# WOMEN'S PHYSICAL EDUCATION
## SHAPING MUSCLE & BEAUTY
### [TRANSLATED]

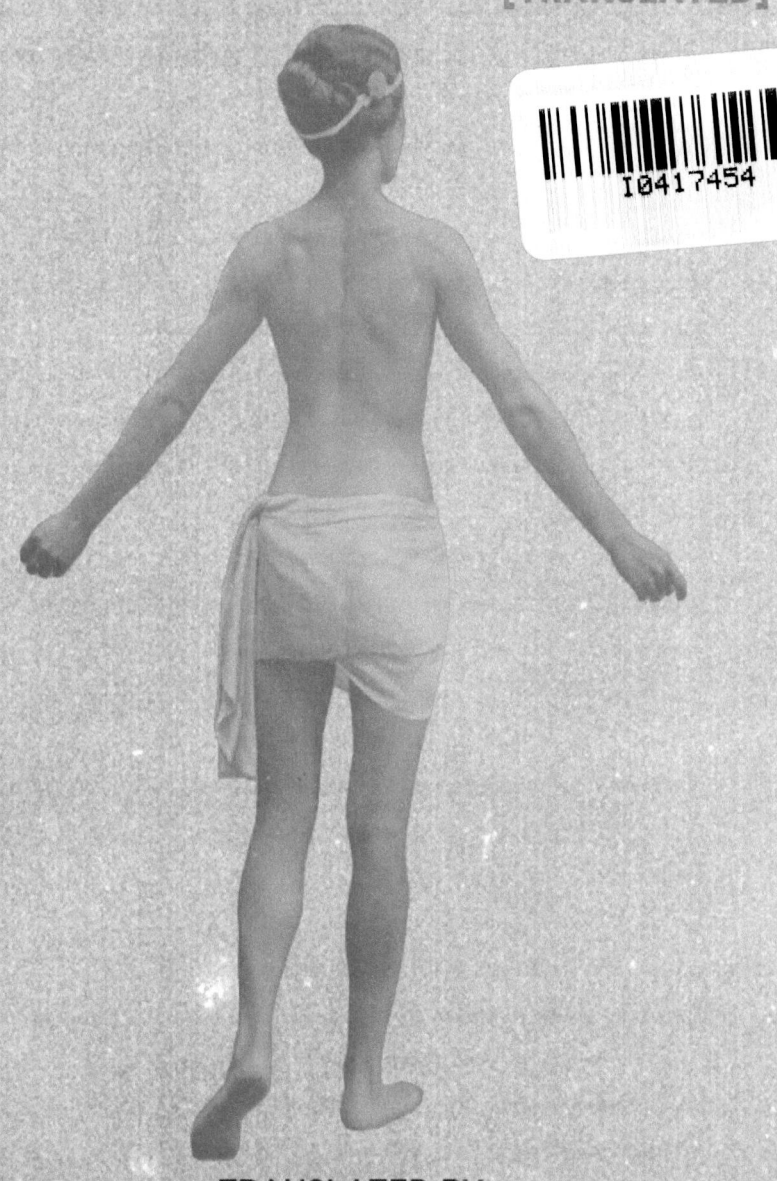

TRANSLATED BY
# PHILIPPE TIL

# CONTENTS

# INTRODUCTION & DISCLAIMER

This book.

(Sigh)

This book, several times, almost didn't get finished in terms of my translation. It's not what you think it is, or maybe it's exactly what you think it is. It's not a fitness book telling women *how* to train. It's also not a book explaining the differences in how men should train versus how women should train.

It's really a historical piece that deserves to be read in order to understand how far we (as a society) have come, and of course how far women have come in *accepting* fitness as not being a gender specific thing. It clearly shows you that the issues we face today were the same issues we were facing a century ago. Therefore, if the issues remain the same, *have we made any progress at all?*

Issues like strength training, distorted fashion trends, objectification of women as "dolls", contraption apparel (a relative of compression apparel), accumulation of fat on the body, weakness, frailty of limbs, being skinny fat etc. Hébert doesn't just point out flaws in women, he does it for men as well.

Sometimes I would not even allow myself certain thoughts, as our politically correct society taught us to be too sensitive. Some other times, I would be ashamed of his writing because of having compassion for my less-in-shape female friends. How I would get past those issues was simply that Hébert would dehumanize us by equalizing the process and ranking us on the same level as animals. If we can judge animals (dogs, cattle, horses) according to certain conformation principles, why should we be so hypocritical as not to apply the same aesthetic standards to our own species? And so he did. Equal opportunity offender, or ultimate level-headed equalizer?

At my deepest core, I had to realize that, well, in many aspects, Hébert was right. Then, I started being concerned once again and allowed the term "eugenics" to enter my brain, which recalled some scary concepts, only to realize that Hébert praises all non-civilized cultures and admonishes our Western lifestyles for being lazy, for hiding our flaws or enhancing them according to the day's trends, where the primitive cultures behave in a more civilized fashion than the allegedly "developed" or "civilized" cultures, exposing a 180° flip from our distorted reality.

Hébert doesn't indulge in fat-shaming or skinny-praising. He attacks both, and only because his viewpoint revolves around the trifecta of health, strength and aesthetics to possess beauty. A pretty face in an unhealthy body without strength is incomplete. By contrast, a woman who is healthy by ways of physical training, vital organ, digestive, postural and any other aspects of health is considered in his eyes more beautiful even if not gracing the cover of a beauty magazine. He is unfiltered, unapologetic.

And that's why I decided to go through with this. I am a mere translator, a reporter whose task is to relay.

Do not kill the messenger if you are offended, and do not praise me if you believe it to be appropriate. It just is. The conformation standards relating to height, weight, proportions, fat accumulation, peak fitness vs maintenance state, or weight management (in either extremes) are clinically defined, as well as represented in art during various eras, which he studies.

Ultimately, Hébert exposes our insecurities (yes, also men's) and tickles our core values, our intelligence, invites a debate, a conversation, which, at the time of publication, is an interesting concept considering how, with the Internet and social media, everyone can voice an opinion, be it a knee-jerk unfounded emotional reaction or a well-composed, well-argued point of view. So, I invite everyone to take this simply in the context of the times it was written in originally, take a deep inside look into your own beliefs, motivation, shortcomings, validation and "conform"/compare to the standards established by Greek artists during the Antiquity. Allow yourself to be offended, or to agree, and invite a conversation, even if with yourself, debating all sides of the argument. We are no different today with selfies or fitness motivational memes across all social media platforms, we just do it or phrase it differently.

In the end, Hébert's thinking was progressive, avant-garde, fearless and holds many truths. He celebrates women, credits our primitive roots, warns against the dangers of a sedentary lifestyle or body dysmorphia created by the media or sexist authors that relegate women to a status rather than a human being. Best of all, he proves his point by showing us his female fitness students, who can stand toe-to-toe with any contemporary female fitness aficionado, without the hype of a short-term gimmicky program or questionable supplements or clever marketing. Although, I will give him this: he is brilliant at pitching his *Practical Guide to Physical Education*, written years prior, as applicable to women as well as men. Indeed, he illustrates his point by saying that men and women are essentially the same, so why should they train any differently? Nice plug, Georges! - **Phillipe Til**

5

# FOREWORD BY GEORGES HÉBERT

This book is aimed at the growing generation: to the young ladies desirous of ridding their bodies of the ails suffered by their elders, to the young mothers who, having understood the full importance of physical education, wish before all that their own daughters become individuals of health, beauty and strength and not fragile dolls.

Aside from rare exceptions, the women of the current generation have received no physical education; they have not been used to the practice of exercising the body. Thus sacrificed, they suffer from the consequences of the lack of development and the trade-offs of insufficient activity. Their health, their beauty and their resilience feel it that much more as their activity is restricted. Victims of prejudice, of which the most nefarious is the contempt for muscles, slaves to conventions or ridiculous fashions leading to the deforming of their bodies or letting some body parts atrophy, we cannot consider at this time converting many of them to the Physical Education cause or simply letting them take advantage of the benefits that physical activity provides at any age. Their minds are elsewhere. Forced they are to live with their incomplete development, the imperfections of their shape and their specific ails, borne of their muscular inactivity.

The new generation, by contrast, wants health, beauty and strength and the freedom to acquire these precious qualities. Nothing will stop the pursuit of such a healthy ideal, to which the future of the species is linked. This book's goal is to facilitate this necessary evolution.

To exercise, to develop one's body, is, for women, a true achievement, both physically and mentally.

From a physical standpoint, certain ailments that the woman believes to be intrinsic to her gender radically disappear. It is one of the most characteristic effects, one of the fastest results from training. In periods generally considered as critical –of which the duration is then considerably shortened- the trained woman is not weakened and can without risk exert vigorous efforts.

Mentally, a complete change of mindset occurs. As her strength grows, she becomes more aware of her value. In order to produce physical labor, to calculate all sorts of efforts, her circumstances compel her to exercise her will and develop her energy, as well as all the necessary actions for the fight to live. She acquires the precious gift of self-confidence.

The thesis supported in this book is that health, strength and beauty can only be achieved and maintained through exercise. Therefor it doesn't rely on natural gifts. One can inherit beneficial traits; but only continuous effort can turn those into lasting qualities.

Upon lecture of this book, it may be difficult for some vain women, idolized by many hastened or ignorant men that they lack many elements of true beauty. Their natural shapes, consequently beautiful, are so ignored that genetic shortcomings, deformed or atrophied features become fashionable. We have seen tightly squeezed waists, opulent breasts, excessively arched low backs, etc. Today, smaller breasts triumph; atrophied legs, deformed calves from the wearing of high heels, are decreed as extra-fine. What an aberration!

In the presence of such errs, how can one speak of beauty? Without the masterpieces of Antiquity, whose esthetic isn't discussed, without certain primitive women whose shapes remind is of this esthetic, without our young pupils who found through hard work and exercise the shapes admired during Antiquity, we would have never dared to write this book.

The models we inherited from Antiquity simply possess normal shapes, which are common in fully developed individuals.

This book will raise much criticism. It attacks both prejudice and convention!

Firstly, it will hurt the ideals that many men have about the female esthetic. Instead of dolls they desire, wouldn't they become fearful to see stand up before them women with whom they will need to count on, physically and mentally?

Then, man will also have against him inactive and not developed women, who will not forgive us for having have exposed their physical weaknesses. The word *muscle* alone infuriates them, precisely because they lack them.

Finally, we are awaiting the raised the shields of our usual censors, who will scream *Scandal!*

We are aware of all this, we know the objections and criticisms in advance. For long, people of sports as well as we have heard those in regards to male physical fitness. We cannot change the status of things without provoking a reaction, however temporary.

But we have with us informed medical doctors, who know that health is never solid and lasting without physical education, without regular training; real artists, thankful for the return of the normal female esthetic; friends and practitioners of all sports who, instinctively, seek out well-muscled mates; women having understood –who thankfully exist- what can be gained from physical education; and finally the rising Youth who wants a better nation.

We want to thank those amongst out students, who, without shyness, agreed to pose for us and generously through their participation contribute to our allow our study of the female form.

These young ladies all have between three and five years of training. We do not have the pretension to present them as absolute models of perfection, but simply as remarkable examples of transformation achieved through training.

They have not been selected upon arrival at our facility. Like many other women, they came with their own dysfunctions or imperfections. Without the training they undertook, their initial dysfunctions would have remained or increased instead of being reduced or gone, and more or less pronounced deformities, like those shown in our sketches, would have appeared sooner or later and would have negatively affected their beauty.

Thanks to exercise, they have regained a normal esthetic, at the same time as they have greatly developed their health and their strength.

We didn't seek out artistic poses with our pupils, rather simple postures fitting the research we are undergoing. Upon study of these poses, our kind readers will take into consideration the subtle misshaping caused by photographic cameras, depending on the position of the lens.

# FIRST CHAPTER : HEALTH, BEAUTY AND STRENGTH ARE THE RESULTS OF INTEGRAL PHYSICAL DEVELOPMENT

## 1. WHAT EVERY WOMAN SHOULD ASPIRE TO.

To possess health, beauty and strength, such should be, from a physical standpoint, the greatest desires of a woman.

These desires are natural and legitimate. Indeed, without health, a woman doesn't feel this physical well-being that relates so much to joy; without beauty, she has a lesser chance of attracting others, she is deprived of certain small self-esteem satisfactions specific to her gender; without strength she has no drive for activity, the smallest effort turns her off. On the contrary, if she possesses all three of these attributes, she owns precious elements of mental happiness.

Health is the proper functioning of all internal organs: heart, lungs, stomach, liver, or intestines, without any malaise of any kind; it's free spirit, the need for muscular activity; it's in a few words the perfect balance of the body and *joie de vivre*.

Beauty, in its broadest meaning, isn't bound to the simple features of the face. It's the complete thriving of the whole being, harmonious proportions, fine shapes; it is both the softness and firmness of the flesh, the superb and full of life twinkle of the eye, reflecting good health; flexibility and grace in posture and movements; in the end, it is whole charm.

Strength is the ability to be able to produce work, muscular power, resistance to illness and fatigue, resilience towards poor weather; it's speed in movements, agility, energy; it is in the end the aptitude to all kinds of natural and functional exercises.

## 2. HEALTH, BEAUTY AND STRENGTH ARE SYNONYMOUS WITH PHYSICAL PERFECTING.

In all beings, the healthiest, most attractive, strongest are always the more developed and physically perfected ones.

This is an observed fact constantly controllable which suffers no exceptions.

Let's take a glance at any animal species, equine or canine for instance. Which, of the male or female objects, generate the most admiration? Always those who acquired, or were made to acquire, the highest level of perfection by pushing their physical power to the maximum. In the equine species, it's the racing thoroughbred; in dogs, it's the hunting group.

The wild animal, despite the challenge of constant battle conditions of its existence, is in general always healthy, strong and beautiful.

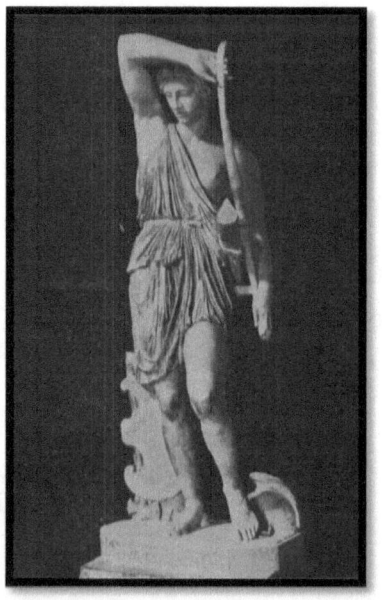

FEMALE ATHLETE FROM ANTIQUITY ERA

Amazon Archer (Capitol Museum, Rome)

Remarkable specimen of integral physical development. Archetype of proportions and refined shape.

The domesticated animal in captivity, abundantly nourished, for which no exercise is possible to fully reach its integral development, remains frail, smaller, without strength and of fragile health, with ugly fur or feathers. It is all the more unhealthy, weaker and less pretty as its activity is reduced, while its nutrition is richer and more abundant.

There isn't anything that illustrates this better than caged birds, when compared to their free likes, or that of poor degenerate dogs living in apartments, overfed but always sickly, without resilience or strength, with atrophied paws and having to wear a sweater to avoid catching a cold!

Human beings do not escape this common law. Certain Human ethnicities are all the more healthy, beautiful and strong, as they lead a lifestyle more in-line with the laws of Nature. It is among primitive or wild tribes that we find the most extraordinary specimens of beauty, esthetic beauty and strength, in both men and women.

Let's finally take a look around us. Who are the people carrying themselves the best, the most alert, those keeping their youthfulness and strength the longest? Always those who, through their lifestyle, are closest to an active life, who are more sensible and do not fear physical effort. A close relation actually links health, beauty and strength, as we will see later.

## 3. HOW TO ACHIEVE INTEGRAL PHYSICAL DEVELOPMENT. NATURAL AND FUNCTIONAL MOVES OR EXERCISES. PRIMORDIAL IMPORTANCE OF DISPLACEMENT EXERCISES.

Humans, like all beings, reach their integral physical development by the simple use of their means of locomotion or displacement, work or comb. That's what can be called the natural law of the development of organisms.

If it were any different, humans would be inferior to animals from this standpoint. Additionally, if scientific knowledge were necessary, the primitive or savage individual would never achieve the apex of their development as a result of their intellectual poverty. However, what do we notice? It is not the civilized, or most educated, but rather, as we already remarked, the individuals of certain primitive tribes that offer us the greatest examples of health, beauty and strength. The latter have received no other teachers than Mother Nature, to whom they have always remained loyal.

The use of natural means of locomotion, or displacement, work or combat are "translated" by the practice of eight main exercise groups: walking, running, jumping, climbing and any sort of progression with the use of all four limbs, lifting, throwing, natural self-defense and swimming.

These exercises can be named *natural and functional*[1].

In the natural life of primitive people, the exercises are obviously not sequenced; they mix and match in all possible ways.

To understand the classification and list of natural and functional exercises, one needs only imagine a human being abandoned in complete wilderness.

Forced to satisfy their basic needs to survive, the human being achieves that both with instinct and any aforementioned list of actions.

Let's follow him *walking* to search for food. From time to time, he will *run* to more quickly reach a specific spot, catch a prey, escape danger, flee; he *jumps*, overcomes or scales all sorts of obstacles he encounters: ditches, rocks, mounds etc.; he *climbs* trees to explore, pick fruits, run away from an animal chasing him; he *squats down*, walks with a bent trunk, progresses on all four limbs or *crawls* to hide or sneak up on an animal or adversary; he *throws* rocks onto other objects, to make fruits drop, hit an animal, to defend himself; he *lifts and carries* his loot; he utilizes his natural means of *defense* (his fists, his feet, his grip etc....) to drop an animal or opponent; finally, he *swims* to cross a stream.

A simple excursion in rough countryside closely recalls all these types of exercises. We walk and we run, we jump on mounds or over ditches, we climb on rocks or trees, we carry food or any other object, we throw rocks and finally, we may have to swim and even at times fight.

Some games and sports remind us also of similar exercises, which makes them that much better. Tennis, for instance, is at once walking and running, jumping and throwing.

It is the *only* practice of all types of natural and functional exercises that allows the primitive human, without any clothing or in basic apparel, to acquire the apex of health, beauty and strength.

---

[1] These exercises can be found in the Functional Exercises (book 3) of The Natural Method.

The requirements of civilized life have created other forms of exercise, other work. None of them are close to replace the first to provide men or women their integral development.

They are either transport exercises to which the body needs to adapt, be it a piece of equipment or an animal: bicycle, horseback riding etc.; or self-defense drills with weapons: fencing and gun shooting; or some acrobatic or entertaining exercises with all sorts of artificial equipment: fixed high bar, parallel bars, trapeze, rings; or games and sports of all kinds, the latter, as we just mentioned, are that much better the closer they resemble natural movements

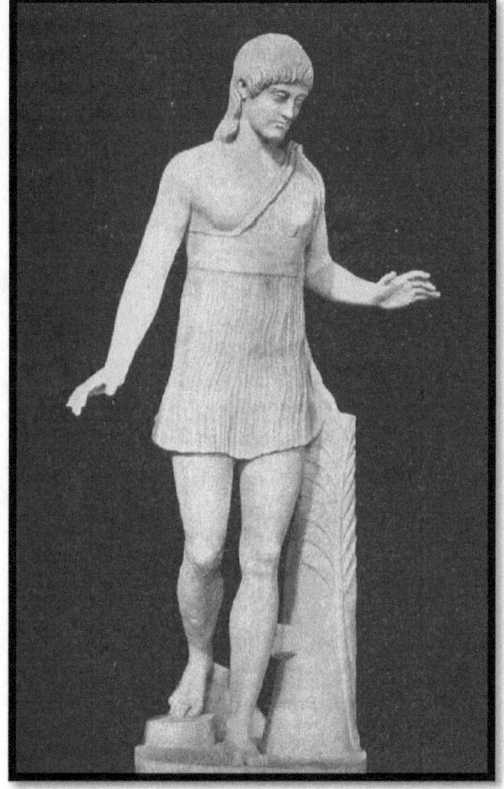

EXAMPLES OF FEMALE ATHLETES FROM ANTIQUITY.

EXCEPTIONAL MODELS OF MUSCULAR DEVELOPMENT.

Spartan Runner (Vatican museum)

Notice the muscular development of the legs, the definition in the knee and pectoral muscle on which the breast is strongly attached.

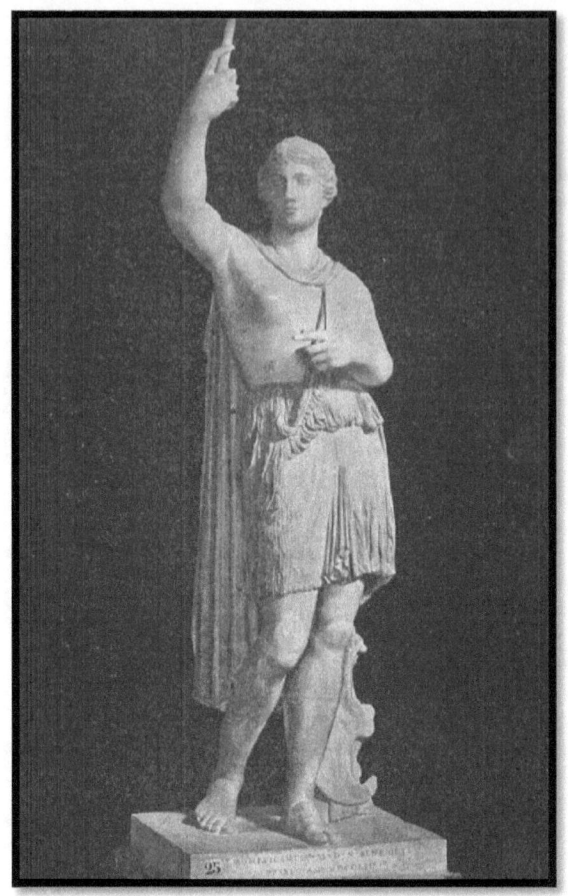

EXAMPLES OF FEMALE ATHLETES FROM ANTIQUITY.

EXCEPTIONAL MODELS OF MUSCULAR DEVELOPMENT.

Wounded Amazon (Capitol museum, Rome)

Notice the muscles of the arm and forearm, development of the pectoral muscle and latissimus dorsi, which border the edge of the armpit, the strong breast attachment, in line with the pectoral muscle.

Functional and natural exercises do not always have the same importance in achieving integral physical development. Observation proves that in all animal species, *locomotion* or *displacement* exercises have priority.

It is obvious that, in the human species, walking, running and jumping or their combinations, meaning any exercises needed to move from one place to another, are indispensable and more frequently useful than climbing, for instance, or self-defense or weight lifting, or even swimming, which is only occasional.

During growth, it is to the process of the fastest means of locomotion that the growing being (child or animal) instinctively resorts to as physical action.

In the primitive youth, much like in the civilized youth, boy or girl, when left free to act, we observe the same phenomenon. Children or adolescents, driven by instinct, perform at any moment, without getting tired of it, in the span of one day, *displacements* at various speeds and mainly seek games where *running* is dominant.

*Running* is, moreover, for the human being, boy or girl, the first and most important developmental exercises.

## 4. INTEGRAL PHYSICAL DEVELOPMENT FOR WOMEN IS ACHIEVED THE SAME WAY AS FOR MEN.

Amongst all beings, the method of acquiring integral physical development is the same for males and females.

Little ones of both genders in any species participate exactly in the same type of activities or movements. What results of it, then? It's that once development is achieved, no difference exists in the abilities of one vs. another. Take for example horses and dogs. Don't mares and female dogs run just as quickly and for as long as their male counterparts?

It would never come to mind for a horse trainer or canine trainer to have special training for women.

Physiologically, women differ from men only when it comes to reproductive function. From the standpoint of physical abilities, limbs, being of the same nature in both sexes, have the same needs and can provide the same amount of work in terms of quantity, duration and quality. Equality here is absolute. The woman is only, physically speaking, the female version of the man.

Experience proves that anything hard that a man does, work or exercise, is equally performed, on any given day, and usually at the shock of everyone in general, by a member of the female sex. War just gave us many such examples.

As last proof of the physical identity of both sexes, let's consider children, little boys and little girls, left to their own devices. It is easy to notice that either instinctively participate in the same type of exercises, work or games, which they perform with the same success and achieve the same results.

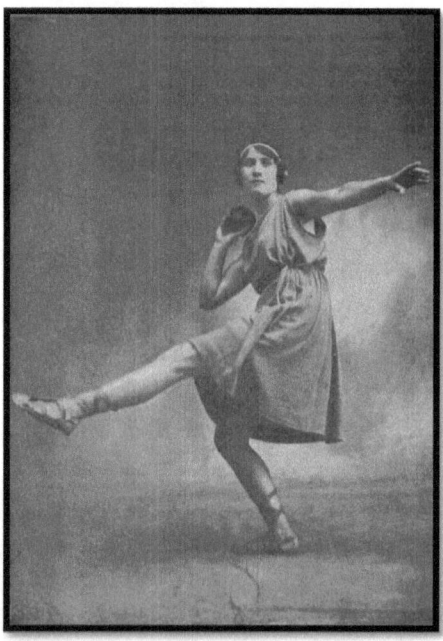

EXAMPLES OF MODERN ATHLETE (AUTHOR'S STUDENT)

INTEGRAL MUSCULAR DEVELOPMENT THROUGH THE PRACTICE OF EXERCISES MAKING UP THE NATURAL METHOD, IDENTICAL TO THOSE PRACTICED BY THE ATHLETES OF ANTIQUITY.

Athletic pose: shoulder throw.

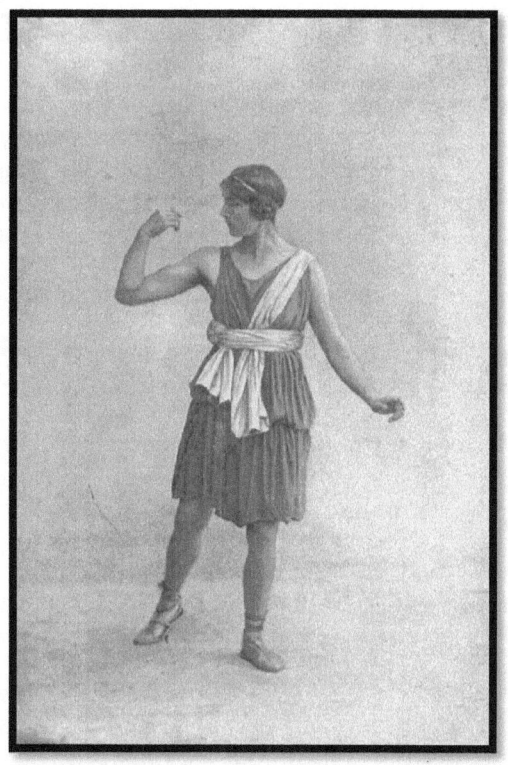

EXAMPLES OF MODERN ATHLETE (AUTHOR'S STUDENT)

INTEGRAL MUSCULAR DEVELOPMENT THROUGH THE PRACTICE OF EXERCISES MAKING UP THE NATURAL METHOD, IDENTICAL TO THOSE PRACTICED BY THE ATHLETES OF ANTIQUITY.

Tentative reproduction of the pose of

"Diane with the Doe"

But, as we will explain later, it is prejudice that makes us consider women like different creatures, physically inferior to their male counterparts. Education creates the differences in physical aptitudes between boys and girls, differences that only increase with age, to eventually become irremediable.

# 5. CIVILIZED LIFE IS AN OBSTACLE TO INTEGRAL PHYSICAL DEVELOPMENT.

Humans are before anything creatures of *air, light* and *movement*. Natural Law is firm: we are designed to live in *open air*, produce *a sufficient amount of daily physical work* (old biblical concept: "you will earn your daily bread with the sweat on your forehead") and *accomplish certain movements*, which we have listed previously. We are first and foremost designed for that.

Civilization may force us into other work; it doesn't change our nature.

The extraordinary speed at which our organism readapts to natural living and the benefits it reaps immediately are all the more convincing proofs thereof.

Any infraction to the natural rules of life needs to be paid sooner or later, and it's the body that suffers the sad consequences: insufficient development, mediocre resilience, muscular weakness, various sicknesses, ugliness, etc.

Natural living remains only the prerogative of certain primitive people. But what happens in civilized life?

Barely born, the little one is swaddled; the baby is allowed to move her limbs only momentarily each day. As soon as she can walk, someone in the family will hold back her discoveries and put the brakes on her natural, instinctive and indispensable activity for her full development, under the pretense that she could get tired, catch a cold or get too hot. Little boys, compared to little girls, enjoy a relative freedom when it comes to movement.

On the contrary, little girls need to surrender from the get-go to criminal rules of stillness or restricted activity, dictated by our prejudice and habits. Playing with dolls is her lot. It is not proper for her to run or race haphazardly like a boy. In certain schools for girls, it is forbidden to the students to run during recess or participate in games involving running. Many moms spend a lot of time throughout the day repeating this perpetual sentence to their daughters: "will you stay still!"

Once she reaches adolescence, after elementary school, a more or less sedentary lifestyle awaits young women. Some begin working at a workshop, office, store, etc.; others go on studying; others return to their families to take care of the household or do nothing at all. Their physical life is now stopped, except for a few fortunate ones.

Most are essentially sequestered. Their physical activity is essentially sealed by putting in place this ridiculous instrument of torture: the corset. Thus imprisoned, stilled and bound at the waist, they will reach adulthood. Why the surprise then that under such conditions, the integral physical development of women doesn't occur?

Their bones will continue to grow, but with deformities (approximately 90% of women having never exercised physically during childhood and adolescence will show traces of rickets or skeletal deformation); their soft tissue develops incompletely or gets surrounded with fat tissue; early symptoms of future ailments appear. Because everything in a young girl's life tends to contradict the eternal law of life: *activity*.

If men were raised the same way, they would be just as weakened and deformed.

## 6. SEVERE CONSEQUENCES OF THE TOTAL LACK OF EXERCISE OR OF INCOMPLETE PHYSICAL ACTIVITY IN WOMEN'S HEALTH.

Women, more than men, suffer the setbacks of modern civilized life.

As a child, a boy can play more violent games; as teenager, he can find, if he wishes so, the ability to satisfy his need for activity (in the sports clubs or gymnasiums, for example); as an adult, he spends several years of his active life outdoors for the duration of his duty "under the flag" *(translator's note: during the then mandatory military service)*. But, a woman, be she a young girl, a teenager or young adult, is always kept away from any physical activity, and even more so as she ages.

What's the outcome of all this? General ugliness of shapes, weakness and even more tragic, an often fragile state of health.

Bad shape can be at least concealed by clothing; weakness forces restriction of activity; but organism troubles are always painful situations to bear.

Good health should be the normal state of the body. In women, on the contrary, as a result of this negative influence of our lifestyle and social conventions, as a result of total abandonment of physical culture, it is almost an exception instead of being a habitual state, especially above the age of twenty-five.

Some women are absolutely convinced that it is normal to suffer some unease, and when one seeks to explain that this pain, if it is the consequence of their inactivity, can disappear or be greatly alleviated by the simple practice of physical exercises, they do not believe it and retort: "It is our common plight, we all must feel something!"

Indeed, what examples are laid before their eyes? Peers suffering as much as them from one ailment or another. It is rare for a woman to not either have sexual problems, which at the very least manifest themselves with painful menstruation, migraines, etc., or digestive troubles (painful digestion, constipation...), or heart palpitations or insufficient breathing when there is a need to move quickly, or simply to climb a set of stairs.

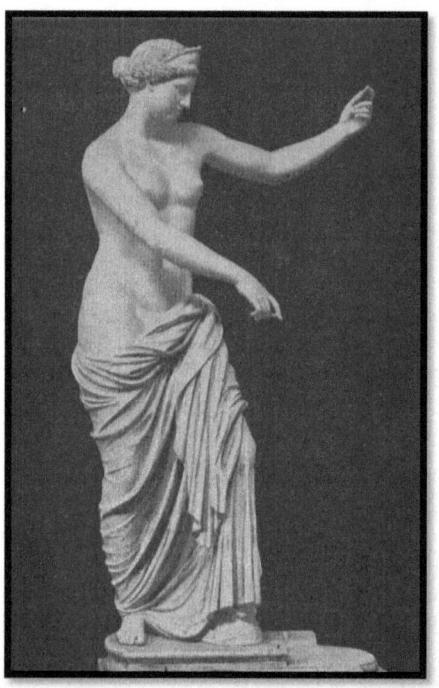

COMPARATIVE STUDY OF ANTIQUE BEAUTY AND CONTEMPORARY PRIMITIVE/TRIBAL BEAUTY

Left: Venus Victorious (National Museum, Naples)

Remarkable example of muscular development of the trunk and arms.

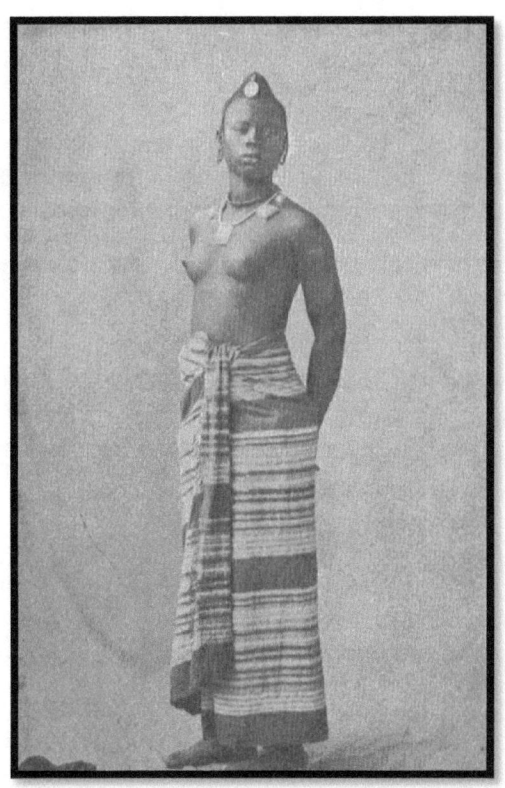

COMPARATIVE STUDY OF ANTIQUE BEAUTY AND CONTEMPORARY PRIMITIVE/TRIBAL BEAUTY

Young African woman

Magnificent trunk development can hold the comparison to the Venus statue to the left. Notice the similarity of the lines of the neck, shoulders, breasts and low back between the young woman and the goddess.

In general, the consequences of total lack of exercise, of incomplete physical activity or of activity not conforming to the laws of Nature (office work, sewing, etc.) are the following:

1) Frequent digestive troubles of all sorts. They mainly come as slow or painful digestion, a heavy feeling in the stomach, constipation, or the opposite, diarrhea or frequent partial diarrhea.

   Constipation is at a high frequency among inactive women, mainly in those whose occupation condemns them to this modern torture: sitting down all day.

   Compression by corset increases or complicates these troubles or causes bizarre ailments. We find, for instance, some women having "flashes" or change facial tones several times over the course of a meal.

2) Periods are long and painful, or irregular. They are announced by pains of all sorts: migraines, stomachaches, low back pain, weakness and even fainting. They cause inability to work, short temper etc. or they last and get complicated, often forcing complete rest.

   The weaker the woman, the lesser the amount of exercise, the harder the period, as a repercussion of this weakness or lack of activity.

   Among healthy and active women, periods are usually shorter, regular, and do not cause pain or sickness. Note this characteristic fact: in primitive women leading an active lifestyle, periods last but a few hours, sometimes lasting one incidence. The inferior physical state of the civilized and weakened woman thus appears strongly here.

3) The heart and lungs cannot bear any *rapid* work, any *prolonged* effort without causing palpitations or shortness of breath.

4) The abdominal belt is always weak and a violent effort, a fall, a jump etc. can cause a hernia.

5) Limbs and joints are fragile like glass, because the bones or ligaments are neither protected nor supported by solid muscles and solid tendons. Any fall can cause a sprain, a strain, a torn ligament or a fracture.

6) The skin often shows breakouts of all kinds: pimples, acne… She has a livid facial tone (the porcelain white look of poets), sometimes even ghostly, which is an indicator of bad dermal breathing or a total lack of exposure to air or natural light. She is rough to the touch.

In good health, the skin is clear, of a more or less darker hue based on the degree of air or sunlight exposure, polished and smooth, soft to the touch. No preparation, no make-up or soap has even been worth good air baths and sunlight to give skin its velvety softness.

7) Sweating or moisture frequently produces a bitter, or fetid, odor, especially in overweight people, despite a clean hygiene. Any effort engaging the heart and the lungs, elimination by the skin increasing intensity, a sensitive sense of smell will easily detect, especially in closed quarters, that the woman producing that smell is inactive.

In good health and active and when the body is sufficiently exposed to air and sunlight, sweat has no odor. The skin has a nice smell.

8) The face's coloring sustains the blow of inactivity or of bad health. It is at times white or pale, indicative of anemia; or red, or frequently rosy, indicative of poor circulation; sometimes yellow or earthy, indicative of the poor functioning of certain organs.

In good health and activity, the facial hue/tint is lively and fresh, but neutral. In other words, there is little or no difference between the color of the cheeks and that of neighboring skin, except immediately after work or exercise promoting blood flow. But in that case, the hue, which is of a nice pink and not dark red, is only temporary.

A very red and flourished, especially rosy, is wrongly considered as a sign of perfect health. It is on the contrary the first indicator of a vascular problem.

9) The eyes, much like facial tone, are also impacted by lack of activity.

   The gaze is dull, faint or on the contrary bright and feverish. Eyes have bags under them, the cornea is stained yellow or streaked with blood.

   In good health, the eyes are lively, sparkling, assertive, and energetic. They are not sunken in and are white.

10) Finally, the body is soft, without spirit, instead of being outgoing and dominated by a natural need for activity.

   If, to the lack of exercise, are added nutritional excesses, other ills appear or complicate those already existing. The most common outcome of gluttony or frequent overeating brings on excess fat, stressing digestive organs and encumbering the body with additional mass it doesn't need. Inactivity coupled with excess food always calls for a steep price, either immediately with digestive troubles, or over time with arthritis in all its variations.

We can ascertain that the majority of pain and sickness due to lack of activity disappears, as if magically, as soon as an active outdoors lifestyle is resumed, that the body produces daily a sufficient amount of physical labor and that, on another hand, food intake is regulated by the work efforts. The war has provided us with numerous examples of this regeneration.

## 7. SEVERE CONSEQUENCES OF THE TOTAL LACK OF EXERCISE OR OF INCOMPLETE PHYSICAL ACTIVITY IN WOMEN'S BEAUTY.

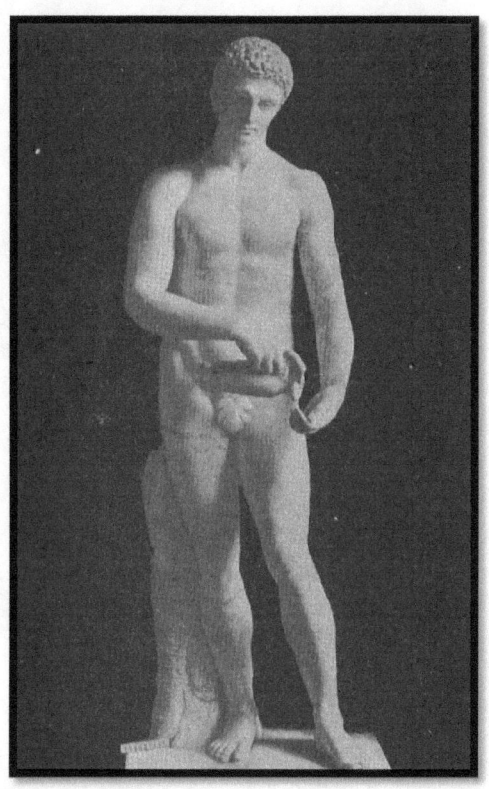

### SIMILARITY OF MUSCULAR DEVELOPMENT IN MAN AND WOMAN

Male and female athletes whose muscular development is absolutely comparable both in power and beauty. Particularly notice the similarities in the development of the neck, shoulders, upper and lower limbs.

Young athlete oiling up (Louvre Museum, Greek marble).

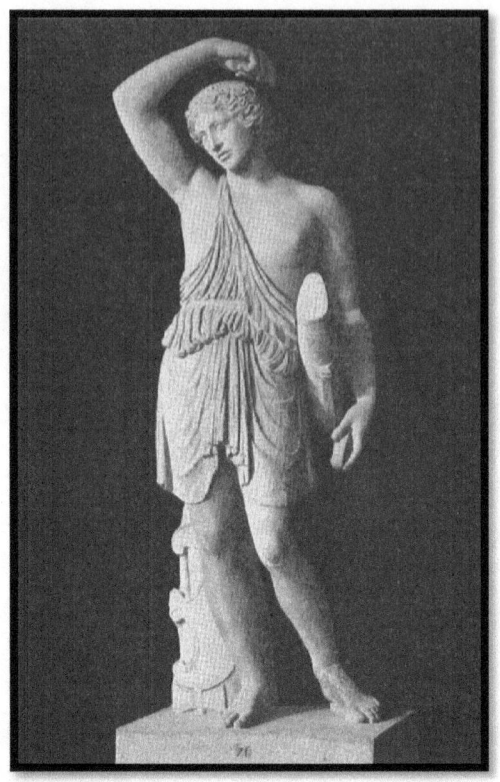

SIMILARITY OF MUSCULAR DEVELOPMENT IN MAN AND WOMAN

Male and female athletes whose muscular development is absolutely comparable both in power and beauty. Particularly notice the similarities in the development of the neck, shoulders, upper and lower limbs.

Amazon by Polycleitus (Vatican museum)

The consequences of the lack of physical development or the state of physical inactivity are not negligible for health as well as beauty.

They can be summed up as follows:

1) In a first instance, *premature aging*, which appears as a more or less alteration of shape. This alteration begins usually around age thirty,

sometimes much sooner, after growth barely ended. That's the price of inactivity.

If women took care of themselves physically, no noticeable deformity of shape would appear before old age; they would conserve the purity of their shape and the advantages of youth till an advanced age.

The facial features, which reflect the physical state so well and change at the same time as the body, would maintain their freshness longer. [INSERT PHOTO]

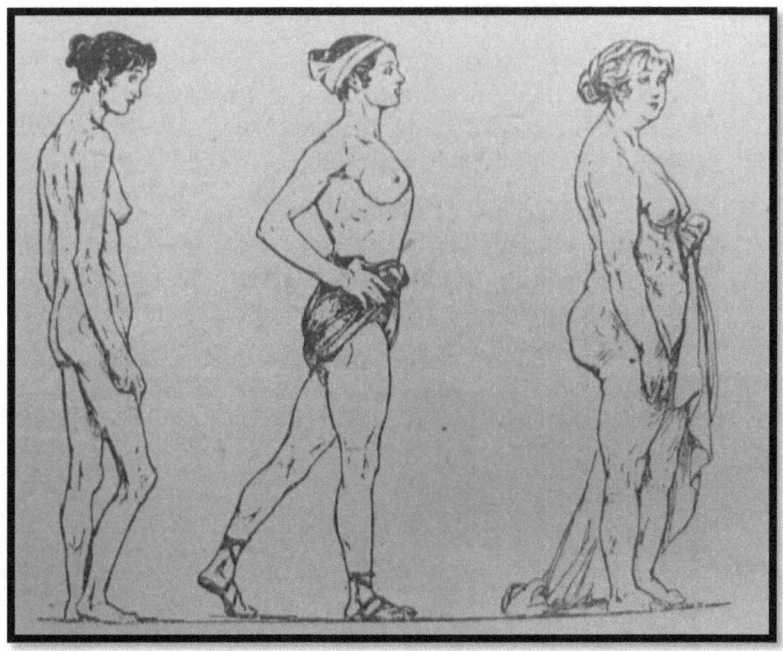

Figure 1.Difference of shape among 3 women of same age. Center: normal type, maintaining her body through regular practice of physical exercises. Left and Right: two extreme types, *skinny* and *overweight*, towards either of which the inactive woman will end up.

2) *Stunted growth*, mainly showing as a reduction in height and a narrow torso. How many women complain of having narrow shoulders and having remained small!

3) *Skinny/waifish* body, characterized by rickety limbs [INSERT PHOTOS], bones showing (visible ribs, shoulder blades jutting out), indentation or abnormal flattening forward of the shoulder, near the elbow, under the knee (internal edge), on the flanks etc.; or on the contrary weight gain, through rounded shapes, limbs like sausages, legs like pillars.

Inactive women belong all, usually, in one or two categories: the *skinny type* or the *heavy-set type*, but more often to the second type. Some who appear to be well proportioned without ever doing physical training only have this semblance of appearance because of a layer of fat covering the non-existent muscle.

Their poor muscular development is thus compensated and hidden and their relative overweight shape doesn't show. But a trained eye doesn't get fooled and still recognizes the developmental lack and the presence of fat, despite the clothing.

There is indeed a very revealing indicator, which helps estimate fairly accurately, and with little experience, the abnormal quantity of excess fat of any person. This indicator is simply the degree of sagging under the chin, to which we can add a degree of plumping of the face and sagging of the neck.

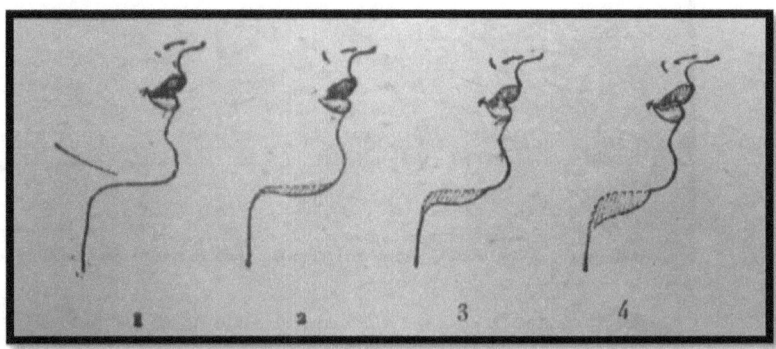

Figure 2. Sagging of the chin.. 1. Normal chin, free of fat. The underline of he chin from profile view is straight or nearly straight. 2. Rounded chin: early stage of sagging indicative of either simple fattening, or excessive depending on the degree of fat deposited. The underline of the chin is slightly rounded and its curve is continuous. 3. Moderate sagging: indicative of fat accumulation in various body parts. The contour line is no longer continuous: a double chin is forming. 4. Heavy sagging, indicative of

localized and/or generalized excess fat accumulation. The double chin is pronounced.

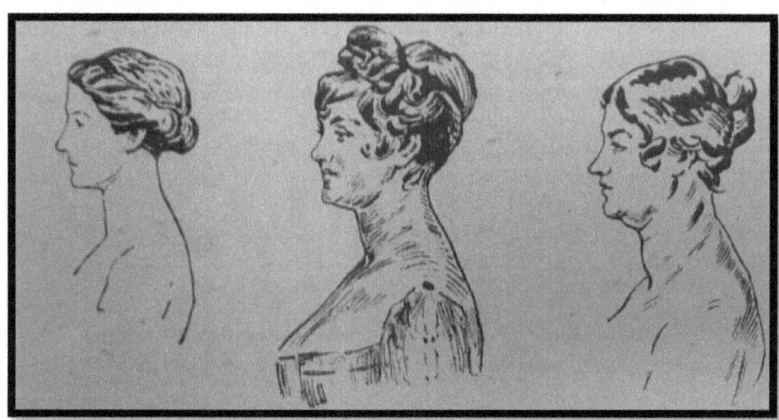

Figure 3 .Progressive alterations of the facial lines and neck shape resulting from fat accumulation. Left: normal neck and facial appearance, free of fat. Center: slight swelling of the face and thickening of the neck, indicative of local fat accumulation. Right: Pronounced swelling and thickening, indicative of general accumulation of fat. Double chin and fat deposits around the neck. Notice that the angle of the underline of the chin is nearly straight on the normal neck, and that it becomes steeper with the progressive accumulation of fat around the neck at on the face.

From the standpoint of perfect development as well as from the standpoint of beauty, the under part of the chin is free of fat, the skin contours the lower jaw perfectly. From the tip of the chin to the angle of the neck, the line, from profile, is straight or nearly straight, but never with a double or triple curve. Also, the angle of this line with the neck's line in the normal carry of the head is at a right or nearly right angle, in a state of perfect development, without fat. This angle becomes wider as food the swelling of the face and neck increase.

A sagging chin always betrays an abnormal accumulation of fat near the waist; it's some sort of record-tracker.

This deformity of the under-chin constitutes a major esthetic defect, but it is so frequent in the modern woman that no one pays attention to it anymore. Teenagers and younger girls already present this change.

4) Spinal column deviations, of which the main ones are: slumping of the back, or rounded back [INSERT PHOTO], saddling or exaggeration of he lumbar curve [INSERT PHOTO], scoliosis or lateral deviation of the vertebrae which slouching of one shoulder [INSERT PHOTO].

Without muscles to support it, the spine always tends to collapse to one side or another.

5) Lower limb deviations:

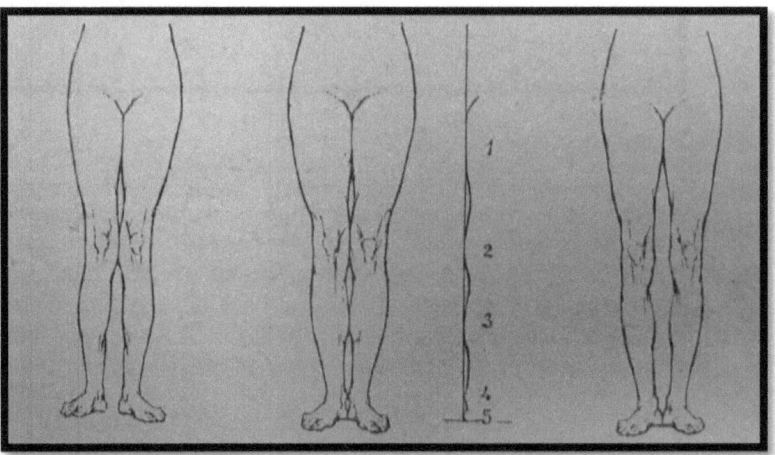

Figure 4. Normal shape of the legs and conformation deviations. Center: normal shape depicting the five points of contact: upper part of the thighs, knees, calves, malleolus and heels.

Bow legs when heels are in contact, or more frequently, knock-knees (heels apart when the knees are in contact).

Normally shaped legs are in contact with the following points, when held together without effort: the upper tier of the thighs, the internal edge of the knees, the internal part of the calves, the ankles (malleolus) and the heels. Oval or diamond-shaped gaps exist between these various points.

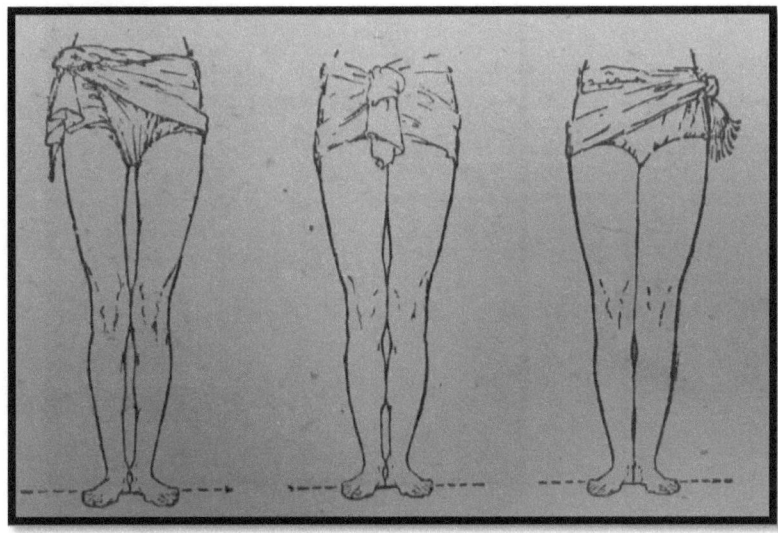

Figure 5.Defective contact points of the lower limbs. Center: normal connection points and gaps. Left: increase in gaps by insufficient muscular development. The calves and upper thighs are no longer touching. Right: Increase in contact points area resulting from either excess muscular development or fat accumulation ("pillar" legs).

6) Upper limb deviations: forearms in an oblique direction in relation to the arm, either forward or backwards. Normally, in full or complete extension, the forearm should be in line with the arm.

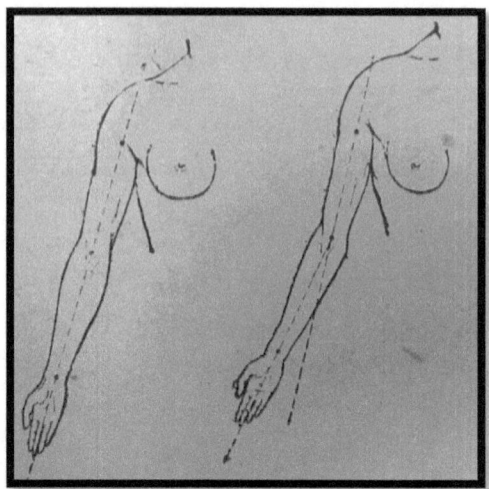

Figure 6. Standard shape and conformation deviation of the arm. Left: normal shape, forearm axis in line with upper arm axis, the arm fully extended. Right: forearm deviation outside the line of the upper arm.

Such deviations are quite frequent among women. This type of extension can make the arm look bad. Thus, many dancers who, out of principle, abhor upper limb development exhibit without a doubt with each extension their deviated arms.

Upper limb deviations, like those of the lower limbs, appear and set themselves most of the time by a lack of exercise during childhood or adolescence. But, a lack of exercise isn't the only cause. They are also a sign of rickets, a consequence of the insufficiency of development from their mothers or simply congenital.

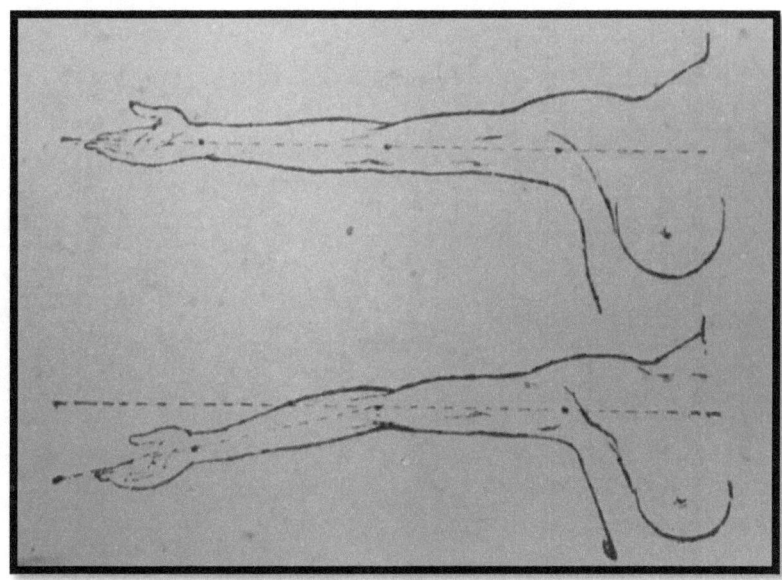

Figure 7. Standard shape and conformation deviation of the arm.. Top: normal shape, forearm axis in line with the upper arm's, arm fully extended. Bottom: forearm extended beyond the axis when fully extended (hyperextension or dislocation).

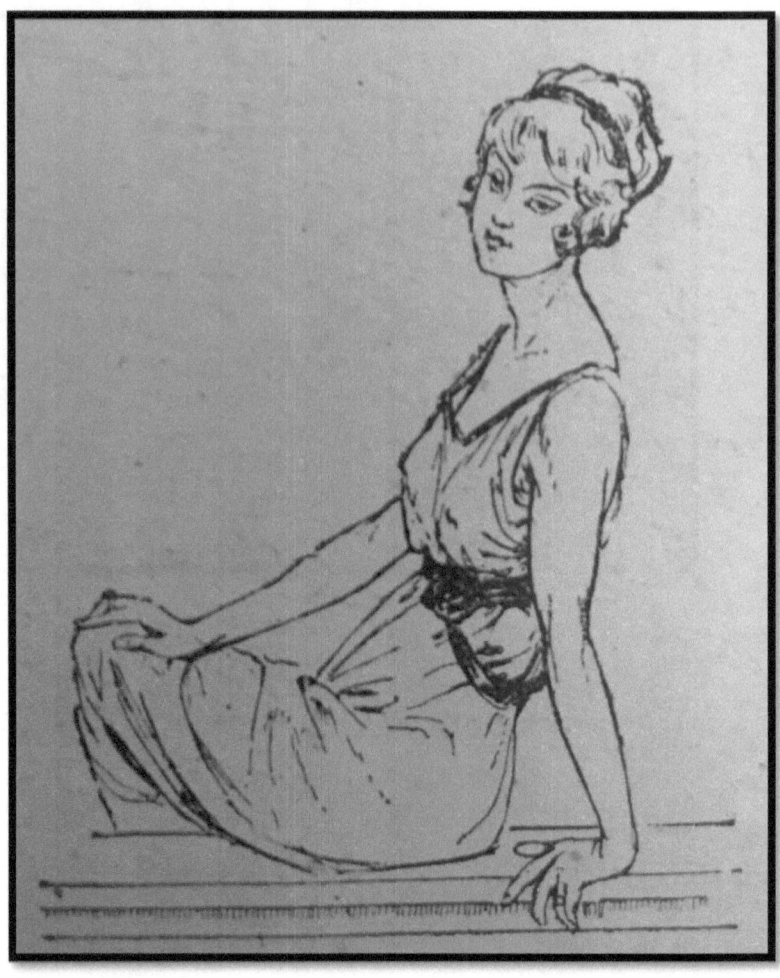

Figure 8.Defective conformation of the upper limbs (hyperextension or dislocation). At full extension, the forearm goes beyond the normal limit and is deviated beyond the axis of the forearm, which gives the arm a double-jointed appearance.

7)  Abdominal drop forward and waist deformity [INSERT PHOTO]. No undeveloped woman, or trained, ought to present a normal waistline.

8) Softening of flaccidity of soft tissue.

9) *Joint* stiffness, betrayed by dry, jerky, incomplete movements or without flexibility; or on the contrary *excessive relaxation*, which leads to dislocated, hyper mobile movements. The *stiff* type and more specifically the *dislocated* type are two types characterizing inactive women.

10) Lack of coordination and clumsiness; forced movement or without grace.

Etc., etc.

In conclusion, from an esthetic standpoint, a capital difference exists between the developed women and the one who isn't. They look like two distinct beings.

## 8. PHYSICAL STRENGTH. ITS CONSTITUTING ELEMENTS. RESILIENCE, FIRST ELEMENT OF STRENGTH. RESILIENCE OF WOMEN IN RELATION TO MEN. STRENGTH AND ITS RELATION TO HEALTH AND BEAUTY.

Physical weakness is usually considered an inherent state to the very nature of women. Don't we often use the expression "the weaker sex" when describing the female sex? More so, isn't fragility, sung by poets under the guise of being delicate, a charming feature quite appreciated by the lovers of "doll women"? To speak of strength when women are the subjects seems like heresy.

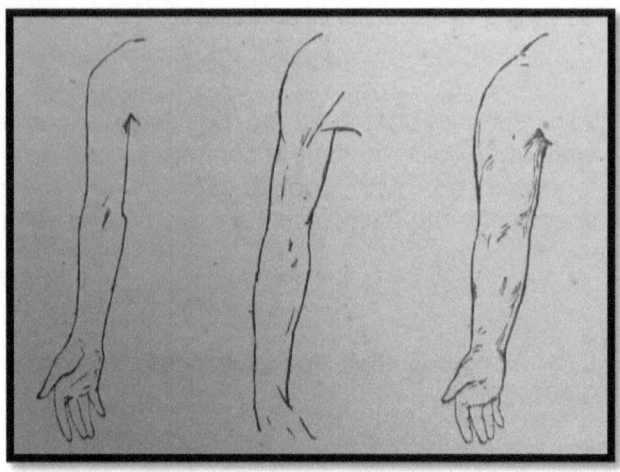

Figure 9. Normal arm shape and its alterations from insufficient muscular development or excess fat. Center: normal arm shape. Left: insufficiently developed arm. Right: excessive fat accumulation ("sausage" arm).

Weakness would have no relevance for women if health were independent from strength; but, as we will see later on, one cannot exist without the other.

We reiterate that women are weak because, as girls or young women, nothing was attempted or undertaken to let them achieve their integral development. There is no other cause.

All the erroneous ideas concerning physical strength come from a false interpretation of the word "strength", or rather a limitation of its true meaning. Here again, preconceived notions are aplenty.

For most people, the physical strength type is that of a colossus, Herculean, wrestler or strongman, or a subject with enormous biceps and thick limbs. However, in real life, what do we observe at times?

One of these men with a reputation for being a solid guy is one day "schooled" by someone of indistinct appearance, sometimes by a "bad kid" or "bad little girl", when it comes to running at full speed, quickly climb a flight of stairs, climb a tree, overcome an obstacle, swim etc.

There is nothing extraordinary in this. It only proves that the one labeled as "solid guy" only has the appearance of strength or possess only a *fraction* of the elements making up strength. Quite adept at lifting a heavy weight, thanks to his mass, he also verifies his weakness or nullity for running, jumping, climbing, swimming, etc. and generally his inferior resistance in displacement skills, in relation to those (male and female) able to surpass him.

Ignorance of the pure or natural type, whom we'll discuss in later chapters, type forged by the practice of natural and functional exercises, consequently is ignorance of the strong type.

The ideal strong type is first and foremost able to produce effort when it comes to walking, running, jumping etc. and of all other natural or functional exercises, displacement exercises taking priority, that type is first a runner and a walker.

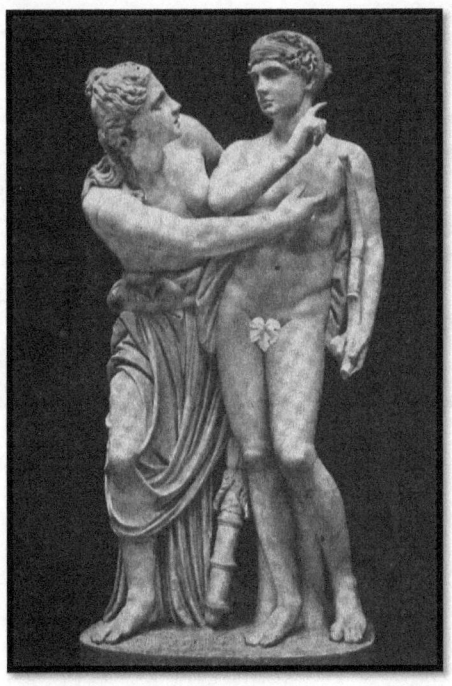

SIMILARITY OF MUSCULAR DEVELOPMENT IN MAN AND WOMAN

Love and Psyche (National Roman museum)

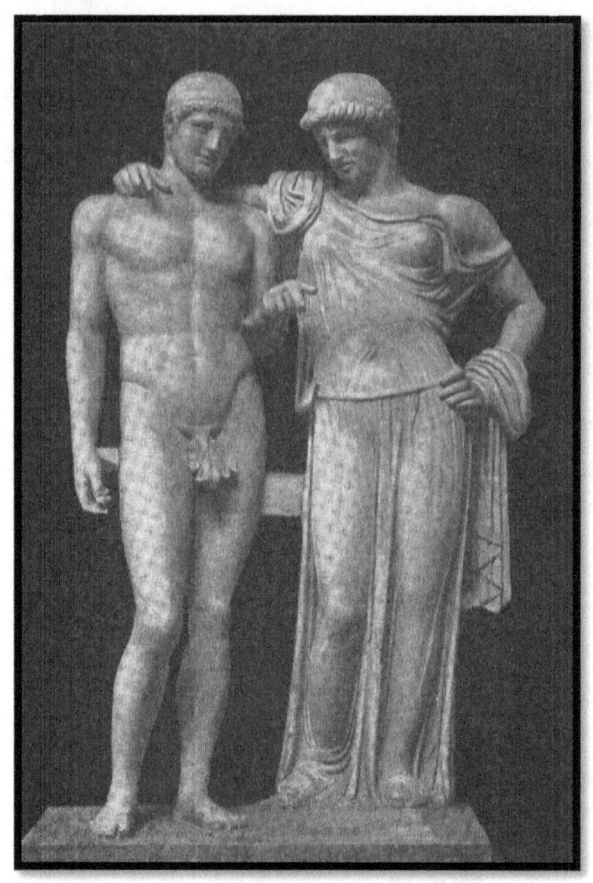

SIMILARITY OF MUSCULAR DEVELOPMENT IN MAN AND WOMAN

Orestes and Electra (National museum, Naples)

Notice, especially in the second photo, depicting a brother and a sister, height equality, with the woman possessing the same muscular development, the same proportions and thickness of limbs, same build, same trunk development, same width of waist and neck, and finally the same dimensions for the feet and hands. Only the hip proportions differ.

Physical strength, in its broadest sense, is made up of various elements [2], of which the most important ones are:

1) Resistance, *endurance* or *breath*, which allow the execution without failing of prolonged work, gymnastics or other, to sustain the same efforts and also to bear fatigue of any kind.

   This element of strength, the most precious of all, depends greatly on the value and function of the internal organs. It is the natural outcome of regular and methodical training, as well as *routine* work of any kind; finally, it also depends on a hygienic and regular lifestyle, free of excess.

2) *Pure muscular power,* or simply *muscle,* which enables the execution with various body parts of sufficient efforts in many aspects: pull, push, squeeze, grab, lift, carry, throw, hoist, hit to defend, etc.

   This element of strength depends directly on the degree of development achieved by the muscles, as well as the nervous arousal communicated by will, meaning the power of the nervous system.

3) Speed, meaning the ability to be able to do quick moves, rapid extensions, spring launches, sudden stops, etc.

   This element of strength depends above all on the more or less high sensitivity of the nervous system, which transmits the command to the muscles to move into action. It also depends on muscular quality and more or less joint flexibility. Long muscles are more favorable to quick actions than short, thick, ropey muscles.

4) Agility, meaning the ability to not only to use one's muscles and use one's skills, but also to preserve strength to postpone the effects of fatigue.

   Energetic, but clumsy individuals generally waste their strength without function or precise goal. They are often, because of that, inferior to those of medium strength who know how to better manage their efforts more adroitly.

5) Resistance to cold, as well as heat and any weather.

---

[2] *The Strength Code* contains the detailed works characterizing strength and the practical tracking of those skills.

6) Energy and any other *virile qualities:* will power, courage, cold-blood, decisiveness, firmness, tenacity, the taste for *action.* Finally, self-control to dominate one's fears under any circumstances, resist physical and emotional pain, etc.

   An individual of medium physical value, but energetic, focused, courageous and tenacious, is always superior in life to an individual having exceptional physical abilities, but soft, lazy, scared and without mental toughness.

7) Knowledge of the process of execution of the *fundamental exercises* (basic educational exercises) and at the same time, a sufficient ability level in all of them.

8) Finally, *sobriety,* meaning temperance and moderation in eating and drinking, and *frugality,* meaning simplicity in choice of nutrition.

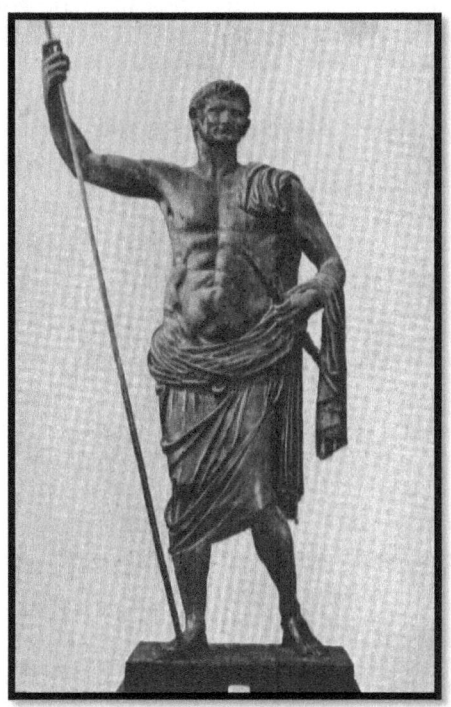 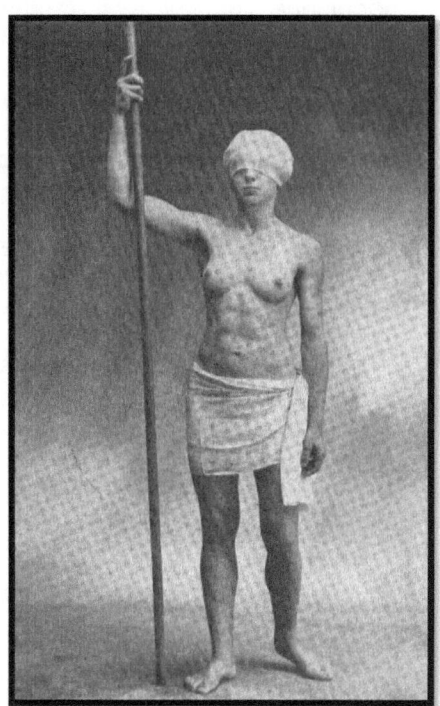

SIMILARITY OF MUSCULAR DEVELOPMENT IN MAN AND WOMAN

(Antique work and modern subject)

Left: Augustus (National museum, Naples)

Notice the muscular definition of the abdomen and particularly the development
of the rectus abdominis, as well as the size of the oblique muscles.


Right: Young athlete, author's student.

Her muscular development in the arms, legs and abdomen is comparable to that of
the athlete on the left.

Of two individuals of like physical value, the one who, to stay in shape or stay conditioned, consumes the smaller quantity of food and drinks and who enjoys simple meals is superior to the other in all difficult circumstances: expeditions, wars, catastrophes, periods of famine, etc.

Thus, to be a strong woman, as well as to be a strong man, it means nothing to have an imposing stature, or to only be able to lift a heavy weight, or to be a champion or record-holding woman in a single discipline or sport.

To be strong is, in summary, to be at once: resilient, muscular, energetic, agile, have endurance, lively, frugal and sober; it's having the ability to walk, run, jump, climb, lift, throw, defend herself and swim.

The degree of resilience, of muscular power, of speed, agility etc., as well as the degree of aptitude to march, run, jump, etc., depend for each person on the innate natural dispositions transmitted through heredity, on body constitution and age. A woman is strong when she reaches precisely her optimum corresponding to her own vitality. This optimum/maximum often varies from one individual to the next in rather considerable proportions. Such and such exercise or easy task for one is a nearly impossible or dangerous effort for another.

Physical strength, comprised and defined in such a way, is in summary only the external manifestation of integral physical development. It doesn't mean it's a prerogative of the "strong sex". Any woman can strive, through training, to achieve its various elements.

Resilience, according to what we just discussed, if the first of the elements of strength. In this particular point of view, many women, even undeveloped or specifically trained, are not shown up by men.

Examples are not lacking, in all sorts of exercises, labors or occupations, be it in the city or particularly the country.

Without mentioning primitive or tribal women, whose physical superiority we already know about, there have always been and still are, even in civilized countries, at times of war, women fighting and sustaining extreme fatigue.

When it comes to endurance or resistance to physical pain, which is a form of general resistance, many a man could follow the example led by women. The opinion of surgeons and dentists is unanimous in this regard.

In the only field where she trains performing the most vigorous and dangerous exercises, in the circus, woman shows no inferiority to man when it comes to virtuosity.

Finally, in the practice of sports, where she is only a beginner, she progresses rapidly; in some, such as swimming for instance, she easily equals man and can even at times surpass him.

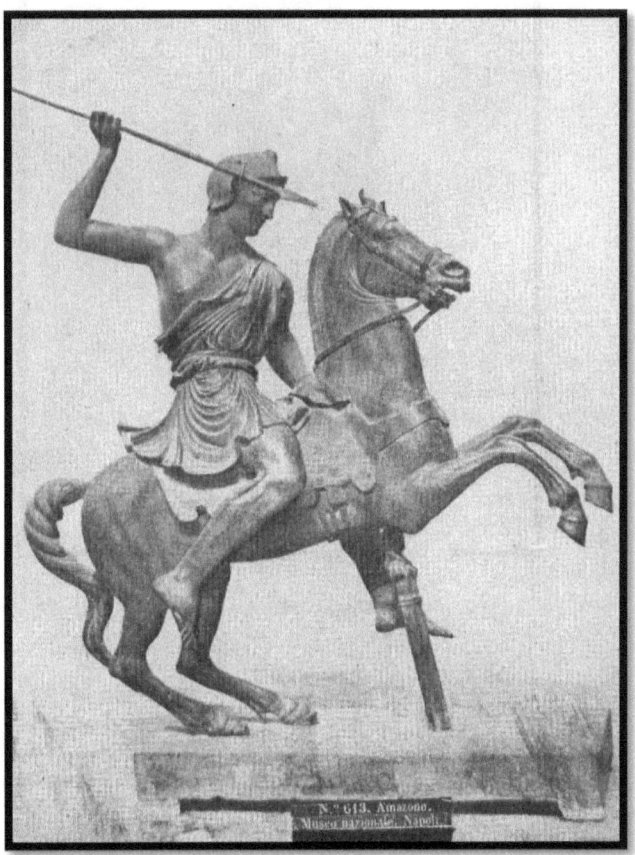

COMPARISON OF FEMALE WARRIORS TRAINED IN THE MOST VIOLENT FORMS OF EXERCISING FROM ANTIQUITY TO TODAY.

Antique Amazon (National Museum, Naples)

Muscular athlete. Remarkable example of leanness and strength.

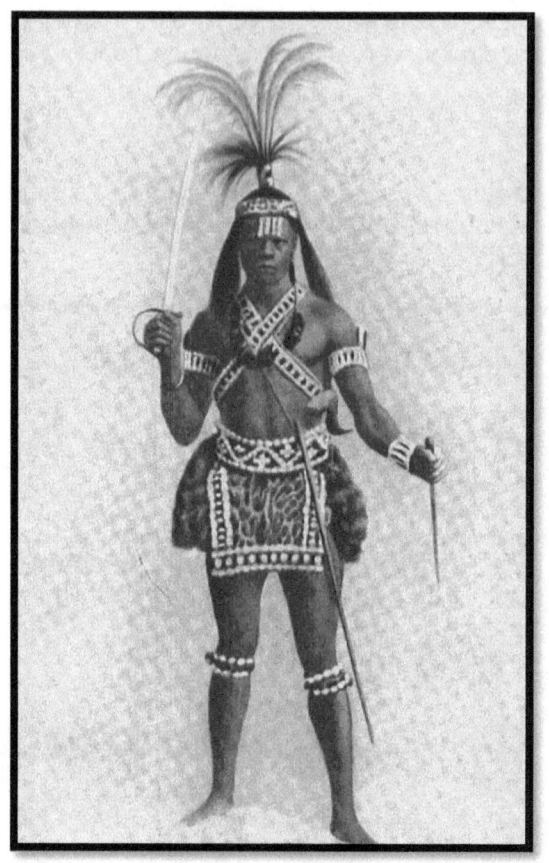

COMPARISON OF FEMALE WARRIORS TRAINED IN THE MOST VIOLENT FORMS OF
EXERCISING FROM ANTIQUITY TO TODAY.

Dahomean Amazon of the Behanzin King's guard, circa 1888.

Notice her superb development in the torso, the shoulders and arms. The breast is
molded onto the pectoral muscle, just like in the antique statue on the left and the
previous photo spreads of Antique statues.

However, it is not wished upon her to fall into, like man, outrageous sport specificity or a professional level, which often cause beauty deformities and health destruction.

## 9. NECESSITY OF METHODICAL TRAINING TO ACHIEVE INTEGRAL PHYSICAL DEVELOPMENT. PRINCIPLE OF THE NATURAL METHOD.[3]

Primitive, wild or savage (*translator's note: the author refers to hunter gatherer tribes as opposed to civilized societies*) beings, as we have described, achieve their integral development with the instinctual practice of natural and functional exercises. They walk, run, jump, climb, swim, etc., out of necessity.

Their existence is nothing but a perpetual physical training session: it's *natural education.*

However, this education remains incomplete as soon as the need to work or to practice such and such exercise ceases or diminishes. The hunter-gatherer, not having to fight to live or eat, as it occurs in rich and calm areas, softens and weakens. Some tribes are thus made up of relatively frail people by contrast to splendid models of development, whom we can find in other more active ones.

Given the obligations of a civilized lifestyle, it is necessary, to reach integral development, to dedicate daily to the cultivation of the body a sufficient amount of time (an hour on average) and to methodically and reasonably perform what the primitive individuals perform instinctively and out of need.

The ideal training session must mirror natural life as much as possible. In other words, it must take place outdoors, with as little clothing as possible, and comprise:

1) The production of a sufficient amount of work, related to age, constitution and the level of fitness;

2) The execution of all kinds of natural and functional exercises: march, run, jump, climb, lift, throw, defense and swim, by allocating to each a degree of importance required and giving priority to displacement exercises.

---

[3] For development related to this method, consult *Physical Education or Complete Training with The Natural Method.*

That is the *natural method*, in other words, the regulated, codified, measured and dosed execution of everything that makes up natural living, for which our body is built and designed.

Before her child goes off to school, the mother must preoccupy herself with only one thing: *to not neglect his/her own free development.*

For that, she must constantly put the child in the most natural conditions possible, and give him/her: *open air* and not just air; *room* to evolve at his/her wish and practice the necessary *displacement drills* necessary for development; and finally, *freedom* to fully satisfy his or her need for activity. As long as the child is a baby, she will not swaddle her so she can move freely her little limbs and thus begin their development.

She must of course keep watch at all times to avoid accidents, but without being overprotective.

The child feels her needs instinctively. Better than any teacher, she knows how to *dose* her work. Without a doubt, she wonderfully applies the principle of *alternating* powerful and moderate efforts. She stops when she needs to and sleeps when her body requires rest.

How sad to see so many moms spend their time stunting their children's natural development, lessening their vitality and deteriorating their bodies by contradicting the need for activity, which amongst children is only the need to live, by restricting or even suppressing its manifestation!

How many congested children, red-faced with swollen cheeks, whose bodies are already overstressed with toxins they can only eliminate through exercise, are pre-destined for arthritis!

The application of the "natural method" doesn't begin when children sit on school benches, meaning the day we restrict on a large scale their physical activity, by forcing them to sit still for hours.

In order to develop, despite these unfavorable condition, a child must be allowed to produce, for a duration limited by studies, a sufficient amount of varied efforts.

The natural method has no other purpose but to ensure this necessary production of efforts and to have children perform, in a controlled fashion, exercises they would instinctively perform, if free to do so.

The application of the method must be followed through the end of developmental growth. The training sessions last about an hour and their frequency varies between three and six times per week. Training gets a particular push for a four-month period, from Spring to middle of Summer.

[INSERT PHOTOS]

Outside of methodical training sessions, young and teenage girls must be allowed the possibility to expend their excess energy in free play and sports.

Once growth has ended and physical development is acquired, all that the woman needs to do is "maintain her condition", which is quite easy, with a more or less frequent and intense practice of various sorts of natural and functional exercises, or through sports, walks, hikes etc., resembling those various activities.

The woman can now live on these acquired skills and maintain good health, beauty and strength till an advanced age, if she can respect at the same time the rules of hygiene relative to the outdoors, proper nutrition, sleep, etc., and to not indulge in excesses of any kind.

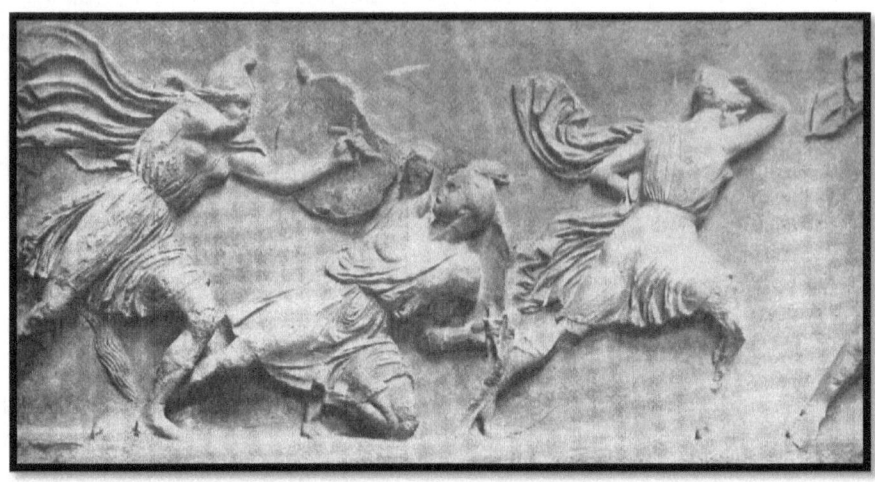

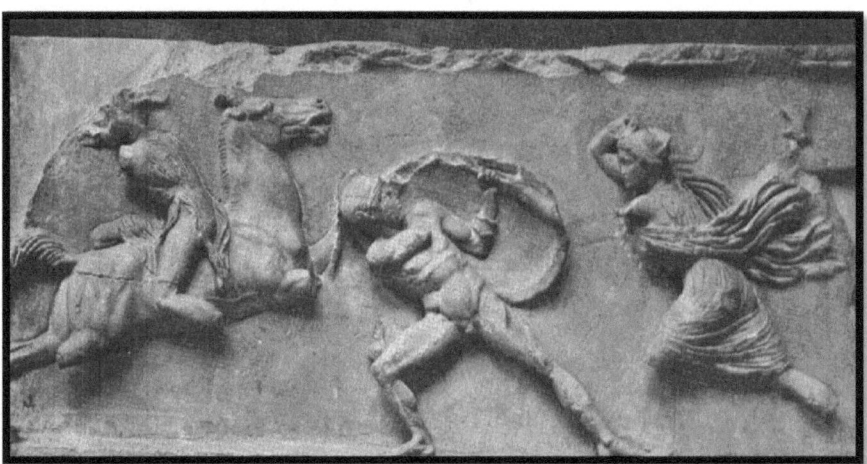

NATURAL OR LEAN TYPE, OR THE IDEAL TYPE FOR BEAUTY

Top and bottom: Fight of the Amazons. Boards on the Parthenon (British museum, London).

Lean athletic female warriors of equally powerful and developed musculature equivalent to the male warriors they are fighting.

# CHAPTER II : BEAUTY AND UGLINESS

## 10.  VARIOUS AND CONTRADICTORY OPINIONS CONCERNING BEAUTY AND UGLINESS.

Nothing is more discussed and given more controversy than the elements of beauty in women.

Both genders do not exactly share the same opinion on the topic. Every man creates, early on, a feminine ideal for beauty, under the influence of feelings for this or that person. His chosen one is evidently a beauty queen. As Romeo said: is there *"a woman more beautiful than the one I love?"*

On another hand, and this is quite human, every woman believes to possess all or part of the elements of beauty as she conceives it.

Men and women are nevertheless in agreement regarding certain preconceived notions, which will be exposed later.

Authors, poets propagate these notions by presenting us with the beauty of their heroines under unrealistic aspects, glorifying fragility and weakness, by describing favorably all the shortcomings due to the lack of development or activity: slumped shoulders, swan neck, narrow waist, frail arms, languished eye, nonchalant gait, bright paleness of skin or rosy tone, etc.

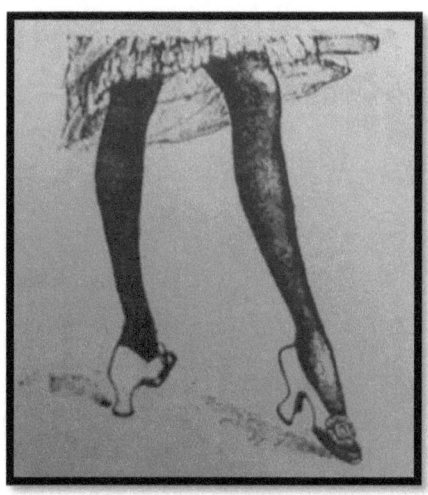

Figure 10. Feminine ideal according to some contemporary illustrators. Thinness mistaken with atrophy.Legs without muscles are "stick-like" ankles without strong tendons have no flesh, which gives the illusion of leanness. Constant pantarflexion as a result of high heels extends the leg line. In such cases, malleoli look overly pronounced.

Contemporary painters and sculptors, having most of the time only models with an inferior physical development, render common the woman type that is incompletely developed muscularly, with round shapes, frail arms, sagging breasts, deformed by corsets, with a swollen belly or with lumps of fat, abnormal skin folds, deviated big toes, etc.

Authors or works on beauty, ignoring the natural or svelte type, which will be spoken later, make us worship, on one hand, male subjects with big muscles, exaggerated by work or strength training (like workhorses) and, on another hand, female subjects without any muscular shape, with fatty limbs, or atrophied by lack of exercises.

Masters patronize publications of so called aesthetic nudes, true collections of horror, which falsify mass appeal, where the ugliness of poses and subjects' gestures only rival their own.

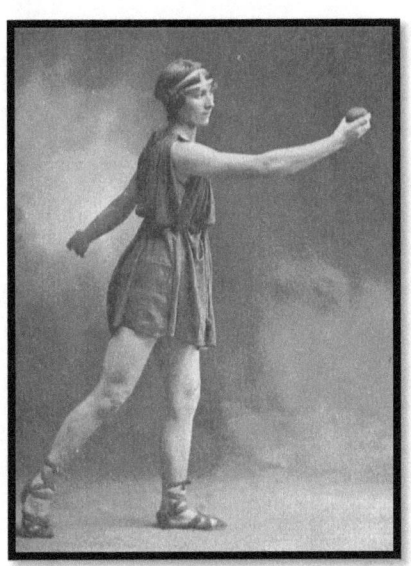 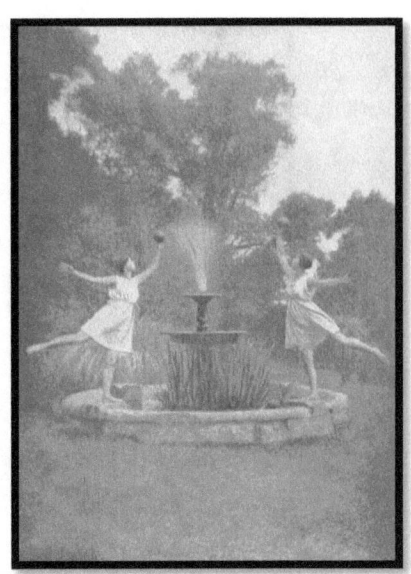

LEAN BODY TYPE WITH LONG MUSCLES

Lean female athletes (author's students) whose limb lines and development can be compared to that of the previously depicted Amazons.

Some common publications entertain with their drawings the taste for "women dolls", delicate and fragile, all head and legs, attired, made-up, invariably planted on high heels, luxury item whose skin no one dares touching at the risk of breaking her.

Finally, fashion drawings, advertisements for fashion designers and corset makers break records of unrealistic deformed depictions of the female body.

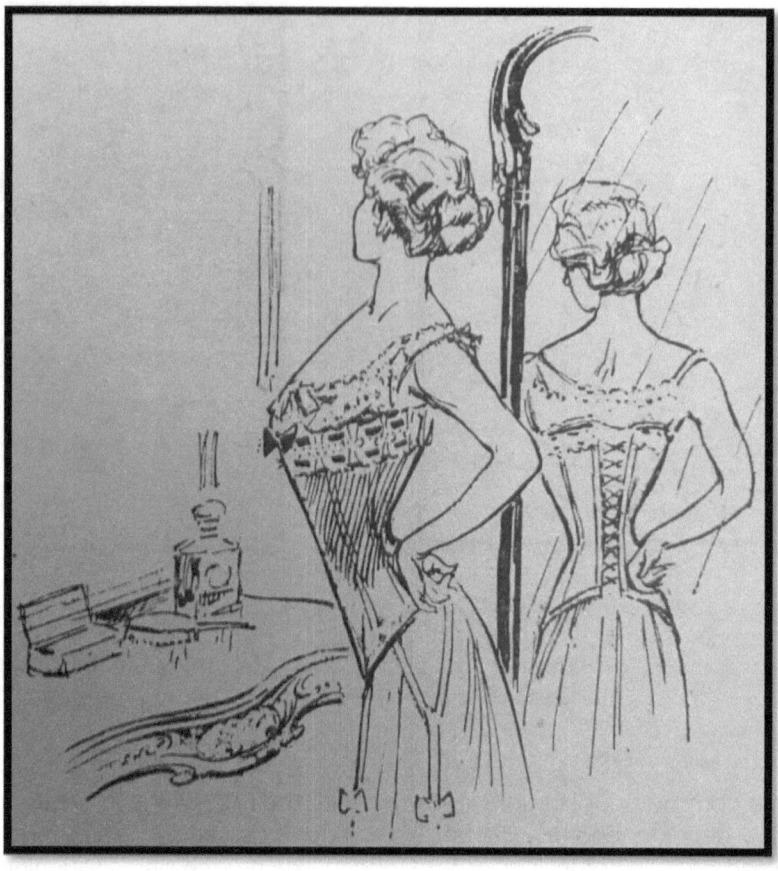

Figure 11. Model of elegance and hygiene! Taken from a catalogue published a few years back. Low chest, arched low back, such were the rules decided upon by the then fashion judges who publicized this instrument of torture. "With this corset, the waistline is deliciously arched" said the caption in the catalogue.

In light of such diverse and fantasized representations of their bodies, how do we expect women to create an accurate idea of true beauty?

# 11. THE ABANDONMENT OF PHYSICAL CULTURE IS THE MAIN CAUSE OF THE CONTRADICTING OPINIONS ON BEAUTY.

Why such contradictions on what elements of beauty ought to be?

The main cause is our distancing from natural life and the abandonment of all physical culture, which have taken away the possibility to distinguish and admire the human body in its full development.

To know how to recognize a beautiful body from an ugly or deformed one is of an extreme simplicity if, as we said previously, we admit –and we cannot admit without falling for the fantasy of fashions o imagination- that beauty is, before anything, synonymous with integral development.

Nature did what it does best. Any being is at the peak of their beauty when they reach the peak of their physical development. One is only imperfectly beautiful if one is incompletely developed. This natural law applies to the plant as well as animal kingdom. We have already established which animal species are worthy of our admiration. Is it allowed, to conclude this point, to compare a woman to a flower? Doesn't the flower seem at the peak of its beauty when it fully blossomed? Or do we admire a withered flower, not having blossomed or having suffered stunted growth?

Another cause of controversy on the subject of beauty comes from the constant hiding, nearly total, of the body under clothing. Here, the delicate question of decency comes in;, however, and apologies to our female readers, physical development has nothing to do with this feeling. *Air* and *sunlight* are necessary for the body to achieve integral development. The human plant, buried under clothes, resembles a plant grown in the shade in a greenhouse.

Clothes don't allow to study the effects of movement, or the play of the muscles, no more than progress acquired during development. Also, they hide from sight defects and deformities, partial atrophy that could be easily addressed if the interested parties or their female coaches could notice easily. Health would benefit form it as much as beauty.

On that topic, we must not confuse prudishness with decency. Decency consists of being proper and reserved; in relation to the world, this is a virtue to cultivate. Prudishness characterizes a state of mind, whereby one refuses to study, speak of or observe the nude form out of principle, even in statue form. Some prudes get offended at the mere mention of the subject.

They would never dare take a glance at their own body to acknowledge any lacks in their development, as they feel like they're committing some crime. In those conditions, no physical culture is possible.

In summary, the abandonment of physical culture, the ignorance of integral development body conformation, the lack of female models worthy of that label and leading by example, prudishness etc., gave birth to all sorts of false or fantasized notions on beauty. Some defects are even granted a certain esthetic value. Only the return to physical culture will bring back a just conception of the elements of beauty.

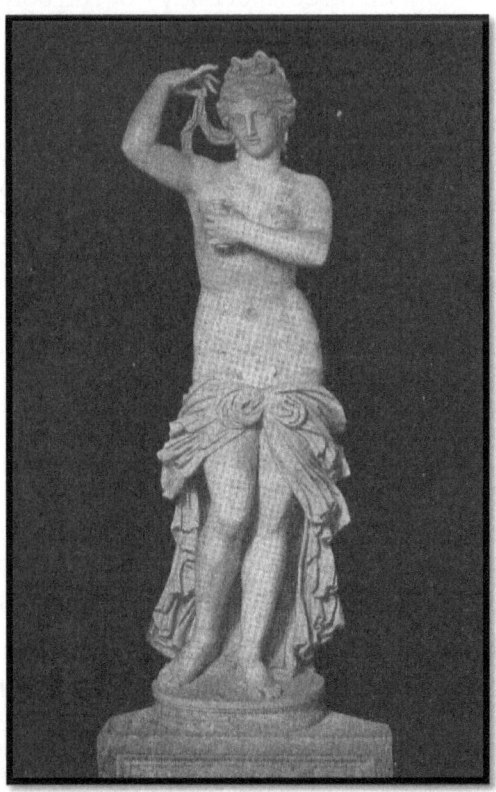

STUDY OF SHAPES IN ANTIQUITY – MUSCULAR ARMS AND LEGS

*Venus oiling herself up* (Vatican museum)

Note the muscular development of the arm and forearm, the shape of the oblique and abdominal muscles, the strong lower abdominals, the waistline. Compare the thickness of the flexed arm, neck and calf.

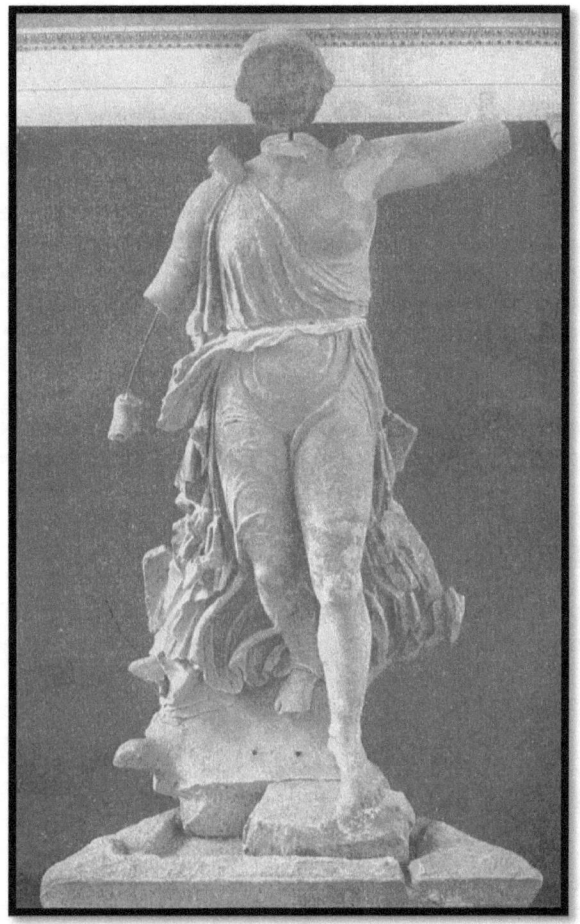

STUDY OF SHAPES IN ANTIQUITY – MUSCULAR ARMS AND LEGS

*Venus oiling herself up* (Vatican museum)

Note the muscular development of the arm and forearm, the shape of the oblique and abdominal muscles, the strong lower abdominals, the waistline. Compare the thickness of the flexed arm, neck and calf.

## 12. PERFECT BEAUTY CANNOT EXIST WITHOUT PHYSICAL CULTURE.

We can affirm in advance, without fear of error, that any woman who has not cultivated her body through a sufficient practice of natural and functional exercises, is not truly beautiful. Among those who never worked, some can be found, well-proportioned and, thanks to their genetics, are in shape akin to integral development. Compared to their less lucky peers, they are relatively well developed, attractively even. They have everything necessary to become beautiful, but they are not in the sense that we infer. That is impossible, otherwise it would negate the laws of activity. Elements of beauty are inevitably lacking.

All that would be needed is to closely examine those who claim to have become beautiful without work in order to become informed.

The first lack that the trained eye notices is a lack of development, either general, or partial, and especially in the abdominal region.

The expression "fairer sex" is gallant. Women are not beautiful simply because of their gender. Beauty is never the reward of lack of activity or physical laziness.

## 13. CURRENT PRECONCEIVED NOTIONS AMONGST WOMEN.

1) First and foremost, *no muscle:* such is the false, most commonly spread esthetic rule. In other words, no normal development.

To satisfy this inconceivable prejudice, women remain atrophied muscularly by voluntarily condemning themselves to inactivity.

How many women have stated: "To have muscles, how horrible! Even for a man; I will stay away from the gym to not become ugly!"

We will later see women confusing thick and fat limbs with normally muscled ones, as well as the big, bulky and short muscles of people in manual labor and strength training, with supple, long, lean muscles, which are the only muscles of creatures of beauty.

Nothing is uglier, indeed, than thick fat limbs or bulky short muscles. But the practice of natural exercises doesn't build this type of musculature.

2) Having a thin waist.

For centuries, many poor creatures, to satisfy this criminal concept, have condemned themselves to deformity with the force compression of their flanks.

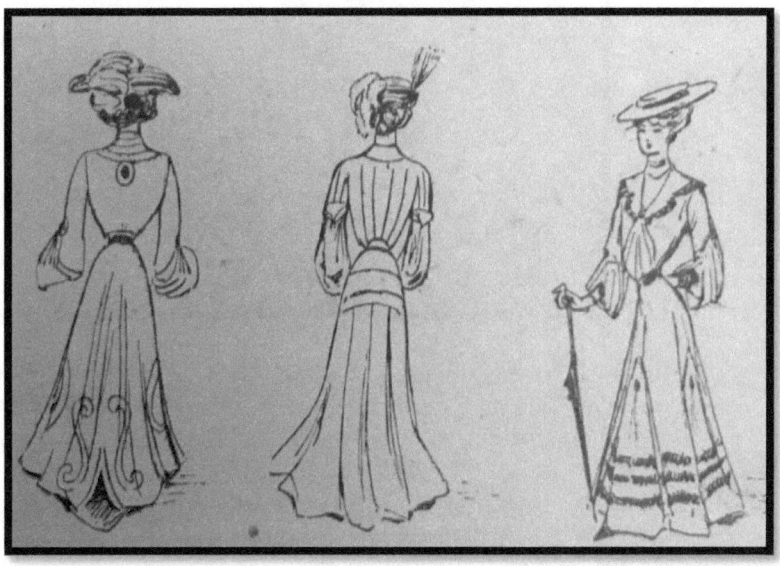

Figure 12. Crazy fashions. A challenge to common sense. Are they women or wasps? Lithographs taken from a fashion magazine dating 20 years prior to publication of this book. All the craziness of squeezing the waist could easily cruelly come back into fashion.

The narrowness of the waist was, even a few years ago, a quintessential element of beauty. Many a man admired this incredible shrinking, which seemed to split the body of the woman in two, and justified this calling it appropriately a "wasp's waist"! Many a woman sacrificed her health for this so-called beauty!

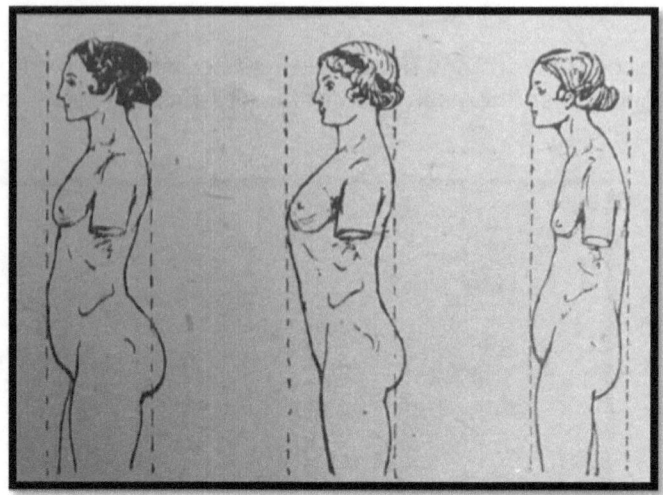

Figure 13. Periodic changes in posture according to the follies of fashion. Rump or no rump, stomach sticking out or in, arched low back or flat, such are the deformations women surrender themselves to to satisfy tyrannical conventions of fashion judgment.

Presently, the fashion for such squeezing is passed, at least for a while, designers and corset makers, judges of elegance, having thus decreed.

We squeeze less, not for health, but simply to follow a different trend.

This may only be a break, and without a doubt, the return to squeezing tight will reappear one day, if cruel fashions dictate so.

3) Having the belly jut out or not, buttocks/no buttocks, all depends on fashion's whims.

A forward belly causes a slouching of the back and a backwards basin, a saddling or exaggerating of the lumbar curve.

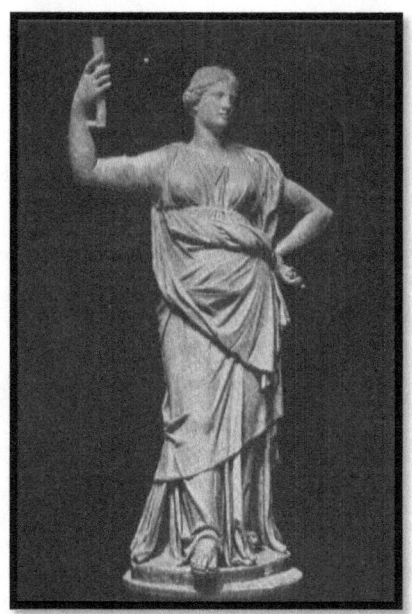 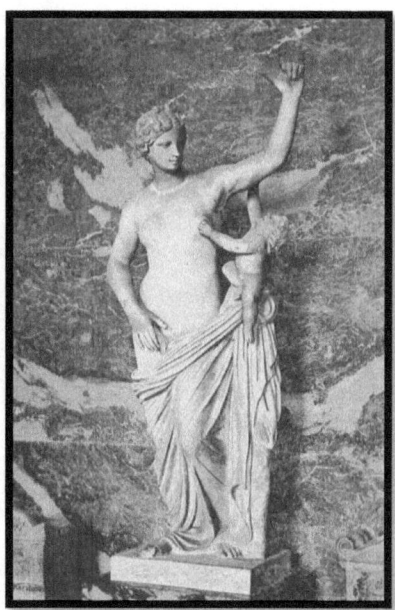

STUDY OF SHAPE OF THE ARMS

Remarkable muscular development of the forearm and arm in statues from Antiquity.

*Melpomene* (Capitol museum, Rome).

*Venus and Eros* (Louvre museum, Paris).

4) Slouching shoulders and a skinny neck.

5) Frail or flabby arms.

A normally developed arm is considered a feature of purely masculine beauty.

Among nearly all women, the shoulder is unattractive as a result of the atrophy of the deltoid muscles.

The triceps muscles, which covers the back part of the arm and gives it its beautiful shape, is nearly non-existent.

6) Rounded calves.

A well-developed calf muscle is not round, an expression that doesn't mean anything anyway. The calf has a specific shape. Contracted, it is like a biceps and presents a sharp shape completely different from its resting state. If it remains round or cylindrical, it is either atrophied or fat.

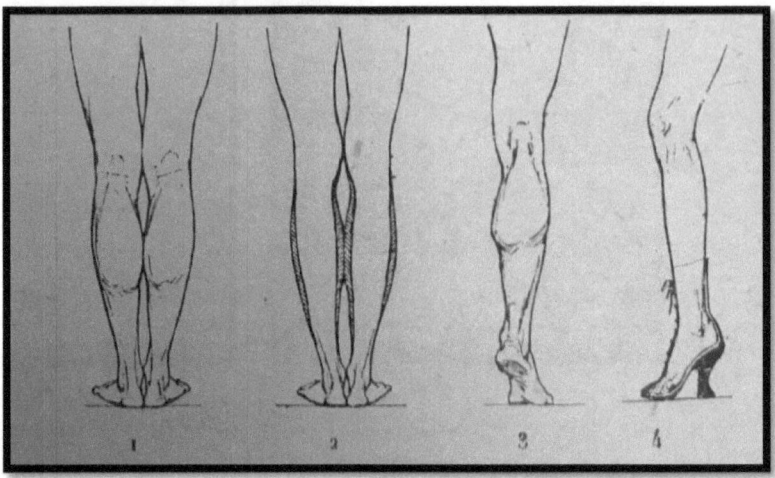

Figure 14. Normal calf and atrophied calf. 1. Normally developed calves, internal edges in contact when legs are together. 2. Atrophied calves: internal edges do not connect. Strong gap above the knees. Legs are like sticks, the greyed out areas indicating where muscle mass should be present. 3. Normal shape of the calf when contracted (with a toe raise). The muscular portion flexes like a biceps and changes from its resting shape. 4. Cylindrical or stick-like leg, with calf atrophy. Common shape in skinny women wearing high heels.

7) Bright white skin, i.e. pale, with rosy cheeks or slightly blotchy (the lily or rose of the poet). We have previously explained the falseness of this notion.

8) Appear tall by wearing high heels.

Almost all women of short, medium and even high stature wear high heels. This manner of wearing shoes changes the natural position of the foot and gives to those who wear high heels a bizarre gait reminiscent of the hopping gait of a chicken.

In a natural walk, *naked* feet touching the ground, the calves or leg muscles have an important action on propelling the body forward. In flat terrain, they work harder than the muscles of the thighs and give the gait its suppleness. Practically speaking, it is never so in civilized countries.

People wearing high heels walk more with their thighs than with their legs, which is vastly differentiating their gait from those women walking around barefoot. With high heels worn by women, the aforementioned dysfunction is pushed to the extreme and walking occurs solely with the thighs.

Indeed, the calf, which during a normal walk has for function to rise and lower the heel above the ground at every step, cannot do so in this case, since the heel is constantly maintained high by the shape of the shoe. With the foot resting on its forward area (ball of foot) solely, and remaining thus fixed in extension, the legs resemble two articulated pistons at the knees and the gait presents the aforementioned characteristic.

As a result of this forced inactivity, the calves remain atrophied among women who constantly wear high heels. The latter explains their round or cylindrical shape. [INSERT PHOTO]

9) Small feet.

To achieve this, feet are squeezed into shoes as narrow as possible, which result in unsightly deforming of the toes, ankylosed toes, callouses, etc.

Normally, the big toe is aligned with the internal edge of the foot. [INSERT PHOTO]

It is always deviated by a standard shoe, and this deviation is so common that everyone, starting with cobblers, this unconscious torturers, believe it natural! Even contemporary sculptors incorporate that into their works!

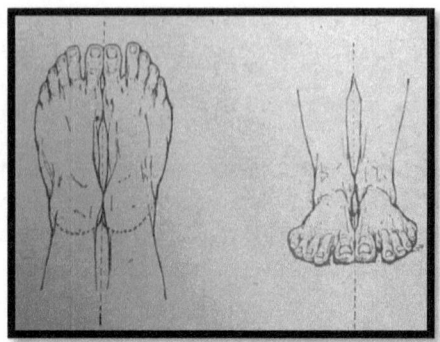

Figure 15. Normal foot conformation. Feet are connected with their internal edges, from heel to toe, big toes touching, with a gap between the big toe and the next toe.

To have normal feet in shoes conforming to the shape of the foot would be considered unattractive, because so rooted are our errors and preconceived notions of beauty!

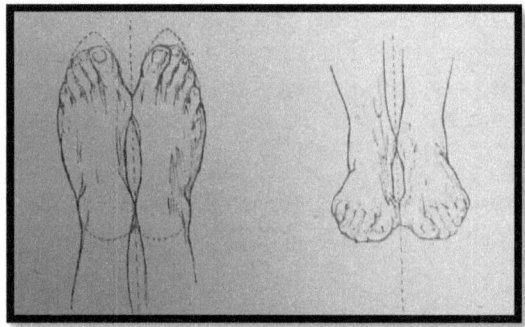

Figure 15.ii Big toes are deformed as a result of wearing shoes. The feet are connected at their internal edges, the big toes are deviated outward. On the left, the dotted line delineates the internal contour of narrow shoes with a narrowing point.

# 14. CURRENT JUDGMENTS AMONGST MEN REGARDING WOMEN'S BEAUTY.

For a large number of men, especially in certain social classes, prominence of chest and breasts, as well as the amplitude of the hips, constitute the two primordial elements of feminine beauty.

It is in general on the volume of these two body parts that they form their appreciation, and for some, their exaggeration, coming from the accumulation of fat tissue or poor shape, opposite of a quality.

The saddling, so common amongst our contemporaries, meaning the excessive arch in the low back, with a pronounced curve backwards of the basin, is not considered unattractive; it is said of a woman with such a shape to have a "nice rump".

A thick and round calf generally has many followers. No matter its shape and curve, so long as its volume and thickness be sufficient.

However, normally developed shoulders and arms, when exceptionally found, are not favored, as they are considered too big and masculine. A skinny, atrophied, round, stick-thin or cylindrical arm, is never criticized.

Feet are all the more appreciated, as they are small. When walking, they are to point outward.

Women who step exactly in line with the direction of their walk, which is the normal or natural position when walking barefoot, are considered kock-kneed!

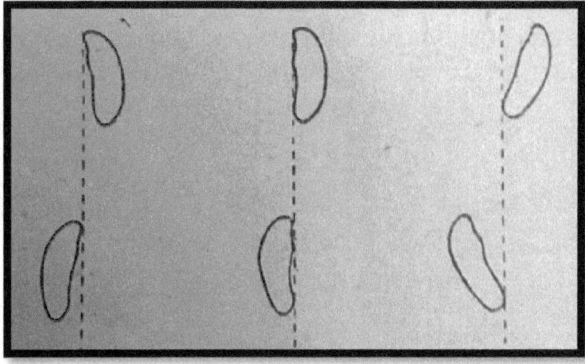

Figure 16. Normal and defective foot position during walking. Center: normal position, the axis of the feet follows that of the walk. Left: internal rotation. Right: external rotation.

In short, a frail arm, a thick calf, heavy bosom and buttocks, tiny foot, aren't those the well-known themes of popular song about women?

Generally speaking, considering the entire body, women with a bit of extra fat, called "shapely", have men's attention, as in this case the fat takes the place of lacking or insufficient muscles, as we will cover in the next chapter.

There is, however, a point on which the majority of men find agreement about women, when it comes to recognize that they should not have muscles, but this I tied to a very specific reason.

Muscle is, indeed, the expression of strength. Jealous of their domination on the so-called "weaker sex", some men, to maintain their position and affirm their superiority, prefer to only deal with fragile individuals, to "doll-women".

To those who physically exercise, men always express the same reproaches, which can be summed up with the following:

- They complain of building muscle, getting deformed and unattractive instead of congratulating them on building health.

- They pretend that women take on a masculine attitude, that they are "turning into men". There are of course women who adopt a manly attitude, but that is inherent to their nature, to their manners, the same way we see effeminate men.

Physical exercise has nothing to do with this. We know some fierce women who never had the need to go to the gym to have a strong male attitude!

However, we can observe that women in the circus, or participating in powerful athletic activities, maintain a stunning grace, harmony and youthfulness for years.

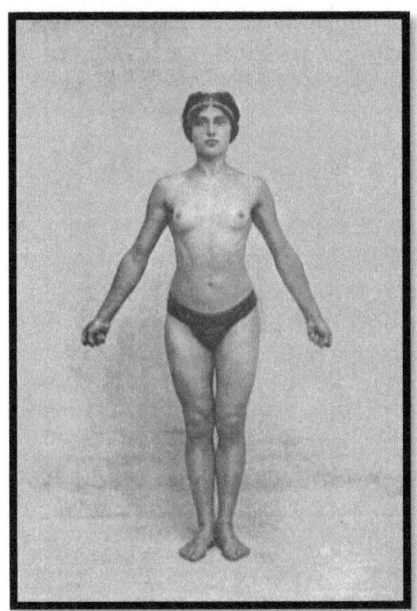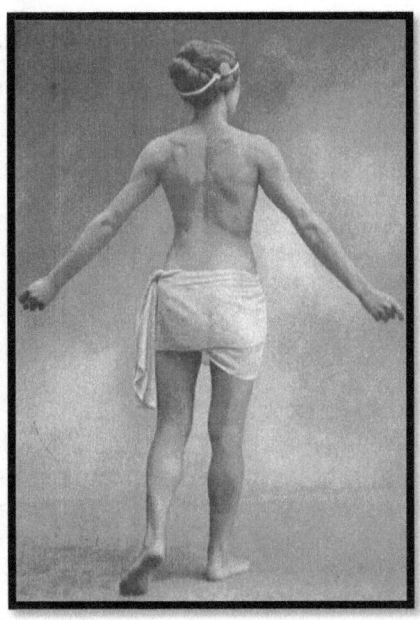

STUDY OF SHAPE OF A FULLY DEVELOPED INDIVIDUAL

(Author's student)

Simple poses allowing the study of the upper and lower limbs, showing the normal conformation of the upper limbs (forearm in line with the upper arm), normal development of the shoulders and back, muscular definition in the contracted calf, a lean ankle, free of fat deposits.

The same ill-will individuals predicting women who train that they will have bad offsprings make the most stubborn of breeders smile. The example of robust families in the circus where having many children is honorable, is enough to prove the opposite. In those environments, it is frequent to see, for instance, a mother and her adult daughter perform together the most difficult acrobatic exercises and being promoted as sisters.

Is it necessary to remind, on that topic, the History of Sparta?

*"To provide to Lacaedemonia (Laconia) athletes ready for war, Lycurgus prescribed training to girls and to let them run freely in public, so that they could have well developed children and they deliver better offspring, expected from their stronger body!"*

*-Philostratus*

Finally, our censors keep iterating this well-known slogan: "women are made for keeping the house and raising children". To which they add this exclamation, which means nothing: "remain women!", but in their mind means: remain weak and fragile, in order to preserve the ideal of the "doll woman". It is always comical to hear such comments spoken by older men.

Notice that it hasn't been so long since the pioneers of the current modern athletic movement have had to fight this nonsense of another kind, but just as idiotic, of the male physical development. For instance, using the pretense of wrestlers or performing strongmen as models of masculine beauty, many people thought that by doing physical exercise that would develop like that too. Writers even thought that a reign of violence would begin, doctors predicted a premature death to runners or cyclists, etc., in other words to anyone who would move.

Nothing proves the slowness of the evolution of our ideas more than the last few examples, when it comes to physical culture.

## 15. ANTIQUITY AT A GLANCE. MUSCULAR DEVELOPMENT SIMILARITY IN MEN AND WOMEN.

There is one topic everyone can agree upon: that of the supreme beauty of antique statues of Greek or Roman women. Why are these statues so beautiful?

Simply because they showcase women being fully, integrally developed and with good muscle tone. Take a look at the *Venus of Milo, [INSERT PHOTOS]* with his exceptional belt of abdominal muscles, her natural waist, her powerful pectoral muscles...; or *Diane and the deer [INSERT PHOTO]* with her jutting biceps, her fleshy shoulders, the definition in her contracted calf muscles...; the powerful musculature of *Flora* [INSERT PHOTO], of *Venus and Eros,* on the muscular legs and thighs of the *Spartan Runner* [INSERT PHOTO], of *Nike of*

*Païonos* [PHOTO]; and finally on the athletic development and of admirable definition of the *Amazons* [PHOTOS].

So? If we can agree on an ideal of beauty, why all this prejudice, this incomprehensible admiration for waifish arms, bony or fatty shoulders, floppy or swollen bellies, which many of our contemporaries exhibit through lack of exercise?

Antique beauty is credited to an integral muscular development, but it goes beyond.

If we compare the women's statues to the men's in like poses, we are immediately struck by the similarity of the muscular development in both genders. [PHOTO]

This is normal and verifies what we said in the previous chapter, when comparing male to female in the animal kingdom. However, the muscular definition in women of Antiquity is a little softer, in some cases, for a simple reason which will be explained in the next chapter.

## 16. JUDGMENTS OR MISCONCEPTIONS CONCERNING RURAL WOMEN, WOMEN OF SPORTS, DANCERS, CIRCUS PROFESSIONALS, WILD OR PRIMITIVE WOMEN.

Why are women living in the country or rural areas, leading a lifestyle outdoors, considered of lesser esthetic, when judging by their clothes?

The previous explanations suffice to understand why these women are not and cannot be models of beauty. They lead an active life, granted, which gives them superior health and strength, compared to their urban counterparts. But it's the kind of activity that doesn't allow them full development.

We have said this numerous times: the basis of this integral development is constituted by the *natural displacement exercises*, more specifically, *sprinting*, to which you can add other functional exercises; all of it practiced in the most basic apparel, a condition to not neglect.

However, *rural women never run*, jump or climb, they do not throw or swim, or get undressed to expose her skin to fresh air or to sunlight, or to go in the water.

Outside of domestic chores, her labors consist of working the fields, which are only slow labors of strength. These strength labors, which we will see later,when exclusively practiced, weigh the body down, deform it and get further and further away from the natural beauty type, built from displacement exercises and speed.

The countrywoman lives in an environment more hygienic than the city dweller; that's all that can be said. But from an esthetic standpoint, she is in worse conditions than the majority of women in cities. A store clerk is, for instance, less active, breathes air or lower quality than the countrywoman; however, she doesn't perform the kinds of labors that would deform her.

Among circus professionals, only those performing acrobatics recall natural and functional exercises (jumping acrobats, tight rope walkers, trapeze artists etc.) have a development that nears perfection. Others bear the specific adaptations to the kinds of exercises performed (weight lifters, gymnasts, etc... who build more mass).

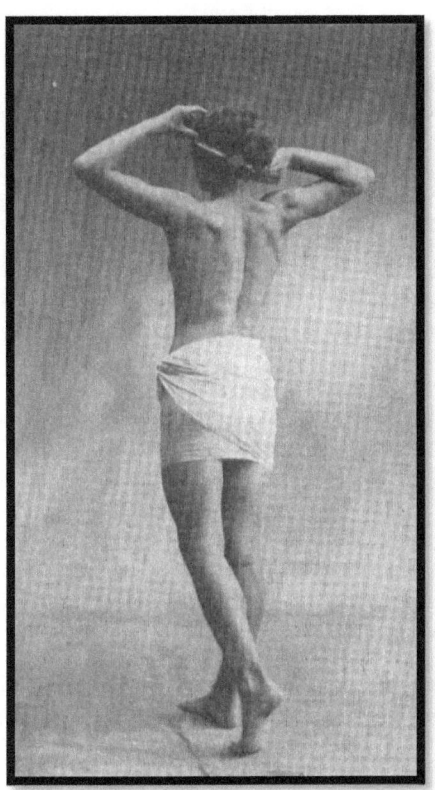 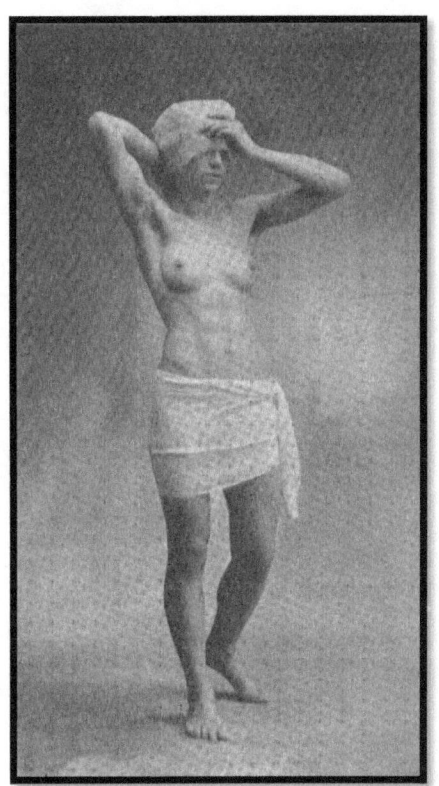

STUDY OF SHAPE OF A FULLY DEVELOPED INDIVIDUAL

(Author's student)

Left: Pose geared at showing the muscular development of the arms, back and legs.

Right: pose geared at showing the development of the pectoralis major and latissimus dorsi, which border the edge of the armpit, as well as abdominals, whose definition is noticeable, especially the external oblique, whose edge is muscular.

Finally, even amongst primitive tribes, many women remain constrained by men to stay confined, or living in near inactivity or complete laziness. They too suffer the consequences of lack of exercise and display the same adaptations or physical setbacks as their more civilized counterparts.

## 17. BEAUTY OF THE BODY IN MOTION. GRACE.

Physical beauty in motion or the harmonious manner to perform a movement constitutes grace.

Grace is also the ability to use all of the body's muscles with ease, flexibility, agility and harmony. It is the opposite of stiffness and awkwardness. Defined so, it isn't a quality proper to women. In men, it is simply called leanness, flexibility, agility and coordination.

Consider indeed a woman and a man performing the same exercise, a single-leg balance for instance. Both do the same movements to maintain equilibrium. However, if both are equally developed and skilled, we will say that she is graceful and the man is simply strong, has good balance or is coordinated.

The reason for this difference of appreciation is simple: it boils down to the physiology of the woman, the expression on her face and also her dress. Naked, with a severe look, she only appears strong, like her male counterpart.

But, any article of clothing, softening her lines, will give her gestures a nearly mysterious value, making the mind work to guess the shape underneath, which produce a charming attraction.

The same way a mere smile brightens everything and distracts the focus from the move itself, which, as we said, differs not between man and woman.

The most typical demonstration of this point is given during ballet, with the performance given by the male and female dancers executing the same moves. What's the difference between men and women?

True grace is the outcome of *simple* and *natural* movements instinctively executed by an integrally developed body. How can one bend gracefully if the low back muscles are not developed? How can one throw and object with elegance and dexterity if the body is untrained, not flexible? Movements are always ugly or awkward when, as a result of lack of muscles or training, they are faked or incomplete.

To be flexible, agile and harmonious, trained muscles are required, then a specific quality achieved only through work. This quality, which we could call muscular intelligence, can be summarized in the following way: to not do any useless movements.

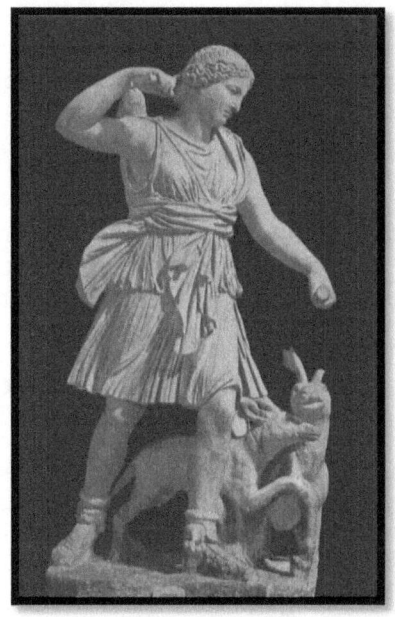 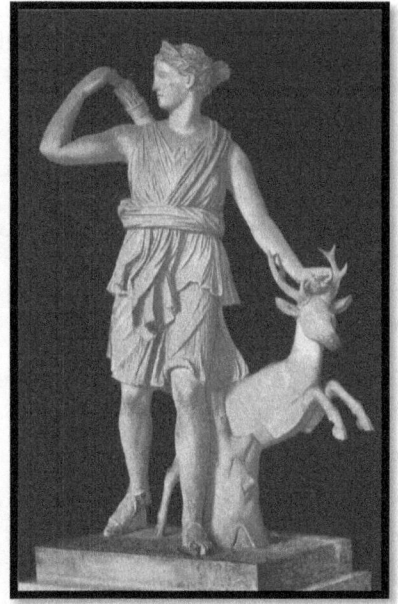

DIFFERENCE BETWEEN BEAUTY OF PROPORTIONS

AND BEAUTY OF SHAPES OR MUSCULAR BEAUTY.

Two female body types with equal muscular development, however differing in shape as a result of difference in proportions.

Left: Huntin Diane (National museum, Naples).

Right: Diane and the doe (Louvre museum, Paris)

Some people naturally lack coordination, are clumsy, and heavy-footed; others on the contrary inherited at birth a good disposition for agility. With equal work, the first group will always be inferior to the second. Some klutzes cannot are incorrigible. Movements are all the more beautiful as they are natural. All movements or conventional exercises, prepared, invented, seem less visually esthetic than natural movements, but they are not necessarily ugly.

For instance, walking with a corset and high heels is of obvious ugliness. The corseted woman resembles a articulated puppet, her upper body in one piece, the basin attached to the trunk.

The gait of primitive women in exotic countries, bare footed and without corsets, is so much more graceful, as a result of the supple freedom of hip movement, something many traveling authors never failed to notice, struck by that vision. It is the natural suppleness contrasting the stiffness of civilized women wearing corsets and high heels, obvious proof that all that destroys natural proportions or encumbers the free play of the muscles, in one word *deforms*, can only produce ugliness.

Take another example: in classical dance, the most beautiful movements are those that appear most natural. By contrast, dancing on tippy toes is ugly, because it is conventional; to stand on pointed toes is unnatural and cannot be done with bare feet.

In modern language, anything called grace is merely soppy, consequence of lack of muscular development.

Movements performed by the weak body of the "doll-woman" are falsely considered graceful; in reality they are only the expression of weakness. Good manners, restrained gestures, even being polite in a teahouse, is considered wrongly to be graceful. A pretty smile, a languish pose, appropriate dress, more isn't needed for a woman to be labeled as graceful. Put this all aside, what's left if there is not movement?

## 18.  NECESSITY FOR ESTHETIC KNOWLEDGE.

To physically educate an individual, it is indispensable to be able to observe, nude whenever possible, the state of their development.

Female coaches and trainers should thus be able to judge esthetically their female students in order to competently track the evolution of this development, troubleshoot, correct or modify the training according to the circumstances and results already obtained.

On another hand, it would be beneficial to the student who is no longer a child to learn how to examine her own body in order to be aware of any imbalances, to be able to track her own progress and also be able to recognize and strive for the attributes of beauty which at once are, let us not forget, those of health and strength. This would be the only way for her to grasp the importance of physical training to acquire a normal shape, as well as of the functionality of certain corrective exercises for development or posture.

Parents should also be involved in the esthetic examination of their children for their greater good and their future physique, health, beauty and strength. How many do actually care? They use the excuse of not knowing anything.

Moreover, it is not in our habits to be informed, on the nude body, of the development of children as soon as they are of age to dress themselves. Next to that, don't we all see people spreading their superior knowledge when it comes to raising cattle or appreciate the beauty of some animal? Many are awarded prizes in tournaments or contests for their dogs or horses, while their children grow frail, deformed, with movement dysfunctions or overweight.

This disdain for a "ragged body" has always been the main cause for our physical aches. Our body, however, deserves our care. It is not just ours; it lives on in our descendants, to whom we transmit our defects as well as our qualities. By not having achieved integral physical development, parents are, in all consciousness, guilty in relation to their progeny. Our children, lame, frail, of fragile health or overweight by our faults, are in their right to be resentful of a sickly heritage.

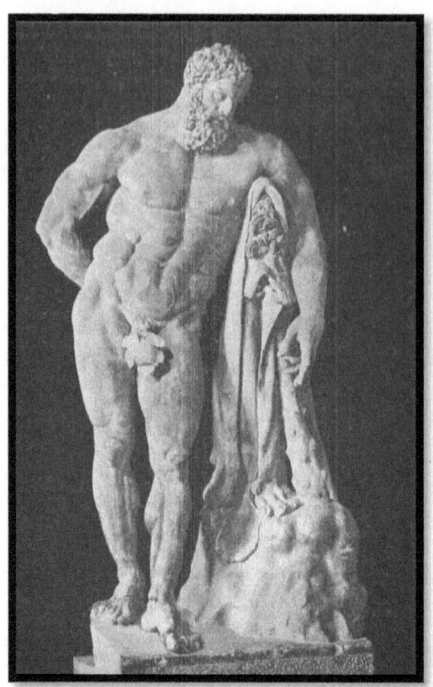 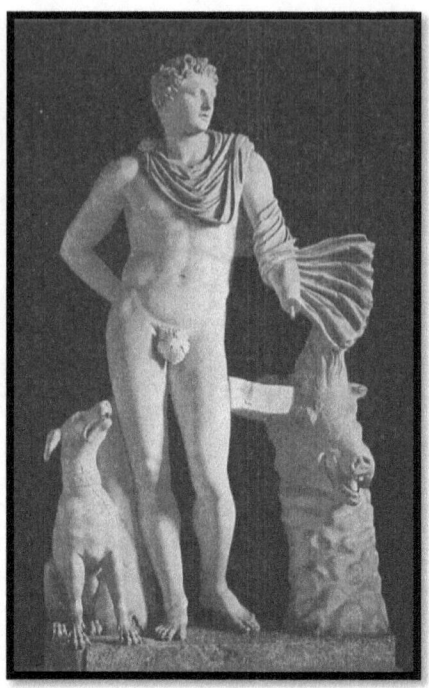

EXTREMES OF TYPES IN THE MALE BODY

THE MASSIVE TYPE OR HERCULEAN AND THE LEAN OR NATURAL TYPE

Left: Farnese Hercules (National museum, Naples).

Heavy or massive type. Deviation from the lean type with excessive work of pure body building exercises. Short and knotty muscles.

Right: Meleager (Vatican museum)

Lean or natural type as a result of natural exercises practice, speed and agility drills, with priority over pure muscular development exercises. Longer muscles of the limbs.

# CHAPTER III : PROPORTIONS AND SHAPES. BEAUTY OF PROPORTIONS.

## 19. TWO MAIN ELEMENTS LEADING TO BEAUTY.

To appreciate the esthetic beauty of the female body, two vastly different elements are to be considered: on one hand, the *proportions* of the various body parts; on the other hand, the *shape* of those parts.

What is meant by proportions is the ratios of height, length, width or thickness existing among the limbs, the trunk and the head. For instance, two individuals of the same height can be drastically different in appearance if one has long legs and a short torso and the other has short legs and a long torso; or if the first one is broad-shouldered whereas the other is narrow-shouldered.

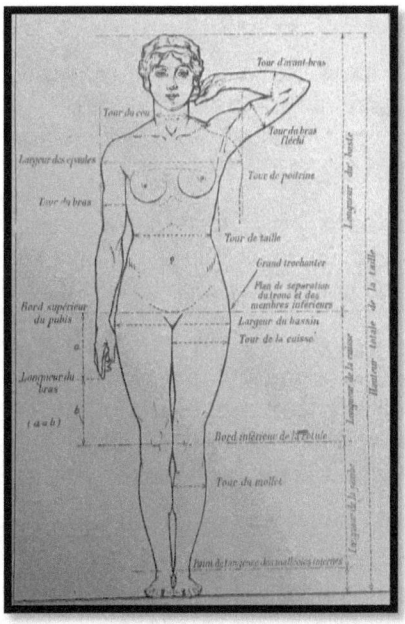

Figure 17. Depiction of proportions and main measurements to assist in studying chapters III and IV.

Shapes are also made up of flesh. They too have a capital importance for appearance.

One person could have good proportions, yet have defective shapes as a result of insufficient development, partial atrophy or excess fat deposit in some areas. Inversely, another person in nice shape could be not well proportioned.

In short, there is the *beauty of proportions*, which relates to the skeletal size and structure, with the ratio of bones between them, and the *beauty of shapes* or *muscular beauty*, linked to muscular development. These two independent elements of beauty only rarely exist at the same time in one individual.

# 20. MODIFICATION OF SHAPES AND PROPORTIONS.

Once growth is over, at the latest between the ages of 23 and 25, proportions are fixed invariably. It is no longer possible, even with specialized exercises, to modify them. By contrast, shapes are always modifiable through training, even till an advanced age.

In other words, it is impossible to lengthen or shorten the length of the limbs or spine, to expand or shrink the bones the width of the hips or shoulders, to modify the skeleton; but we can always increase fully developed muscles, reduce or get rid of excess fat.

This remark is necessary, because some people believe that there are exercises out there that can change proportions. Too tall, for instance, and they wish to be shorter; too short, they wish to be taller.

Before the skeleton sets completely, more particularly during childhood than adolescence, some exercises can influence proportions, even trunk length; nutrition, living conditions and the environment have a serious influence. The science of physical education, or in this case more precisely the science of human rearing, only presents vague data on this topic.

All that we know from observation and analysis, is that strength training exercises, practiced exclusively or in excess from a young age, tend to shorten the child's height by speeding up ossification. And still, this rule is not rigorous, since there are strength workers, gymnasts, weight lifters who are quite tall. Overtraining and malnutrition seem to be the determining factor of the short stature of some gymnasts, acrobats, manual labor workers, etc.

Genetics, in all cases, are the biggest factor. It is illusory to want to stop growth in height as it is to want to increase it in people who are predestined to be either tall or short.

Devices to grow taller are in the realm of snake oil. All that they can deliver is the illusion of being taller, by straightening up a person's hunched posture, but without changing the actual length of the spine or of their lower limbs.

We must learn to accept and live the proportions we inherited. But, what we can acquire through methodical work is the *improvement of our shapes*, meaning *muscular beauty*. Poor proportions, even noticeable ones, can be barely noticeable when the musculature is well-developed.

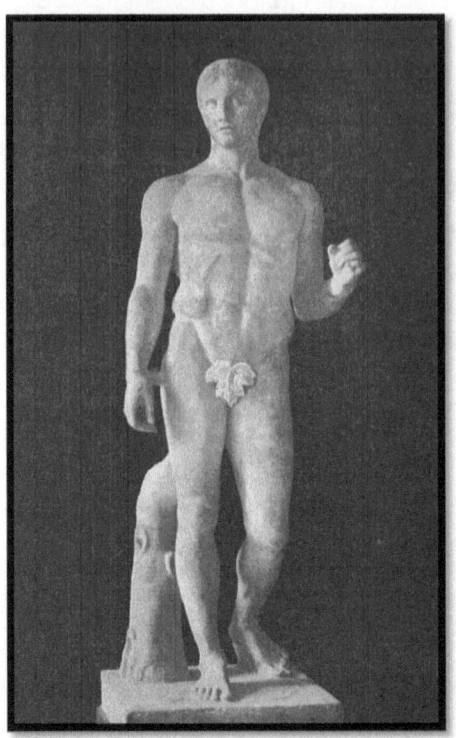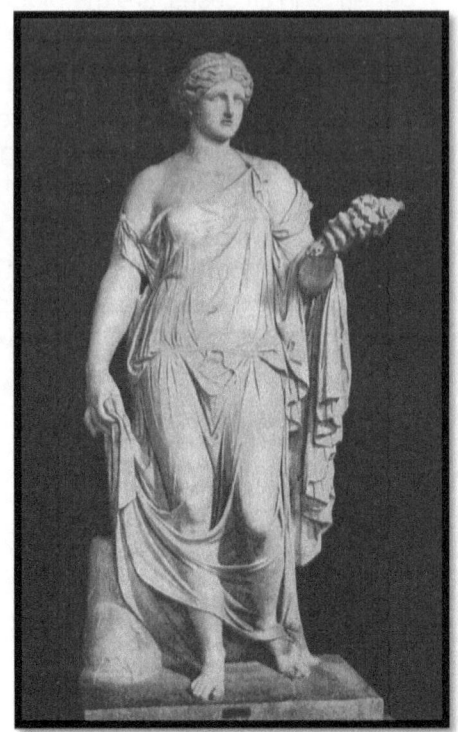

MEDIUM OR IN-BETWEEN MASSIVE AND LEAN TYPES.

Left: Doruphoros (spear carrier, National museum, Naples)

Powerful type, semi-lean, semi-massive, serving as comparison to the Flora next to him in the layout above. Notice the pectoral development in both sexes, displaying the same definition near the armpit, as well as the development of the oblique muscles and abdominals with a muscular lower belly contour.

Right: Farnese Flora (National museum, Naples)

Notice the neck and shoulder line, the shoulder's shape, the suprasternal notch, visibility of clavicles under the skin, the definition in the pectoral-deltoid line, the development of the upper arm and forearm etc. All comparable to the spear carrier. The power of the muscular development of the goddess doesn't take away from her grace or gait.

## 21. HARMONIOUS PROPORTIONS AND DYSFUNCTIONAL PROPORTIONS.

There is no such thing as a standard for normal proportions.

Each ethnicity, as well as each individual, possesses, indeed, specific traits, which are the consequence of their lifestyle, their nutrition during growth, their work or physical training, the country in which they live from a land configuration standpoint, climate or resources. Thus the mountaineer isn't built like one living in flat lands; black people present structural differences from white people; strength workers (construction workers, movers) do not have the same build as runners (like Arab desert runners, rickshaw operators, etc.). Asians tend to be of shorter stature; Patagonians of higher stature; Latin cultures tend to have shorter legs whereas Anglo-Saxons tend to have longer legs; etc.

On the other hand, art and physiology still disagree on the ideal "canon", meaning proportions which are both beautiful and rational.

There are proportions which we could consider "standard" because they give the whole body an obvious harmony and at once provide the ability to do all kinds or natural and functional exercises. That means there are less attractive builds, other can be more or less harmonious, while others still near perfection, i.e. uniform proportions, which will be indicated later.

Outside of a certain limit, there are abnormal, non-esthetic or defective proportions, which not only cause an ugly appearance, but also reduce ability to perform certain exercises. For instance, short-legged individuals with a long torso are not favorable to jumping exercises; those with a bigger build are at a disadvantage for running and speed drills, etc.

In summary, proportion defects come from various causes, of which the main ones are:

- Genetics (passed on by the parents);

- Deforming exercises or work performed during childhood or adolescence;

- Mistakes in physical education;

- Deforming articles of clothing, which squeeze the body excessively (corsets, belts, shoes);

- ◉ Poor nutrition, especially during early childhood (bottle-raised children with bad milk);

- ◉ Overworking in all its forms, during childhood and adolescence.

# 22. CHARACTERISTICS OF REGULAR PROPORTIONS.

The characteristics of regular proportions, despite the impossibility of being able to modify them, remain useful to identify because they give an accurate idea of the conformation of the body. Also, they allow the immediate discovery of any structural deviations of poorly built individuals. We will only indicate the characteristics of principal proportions.

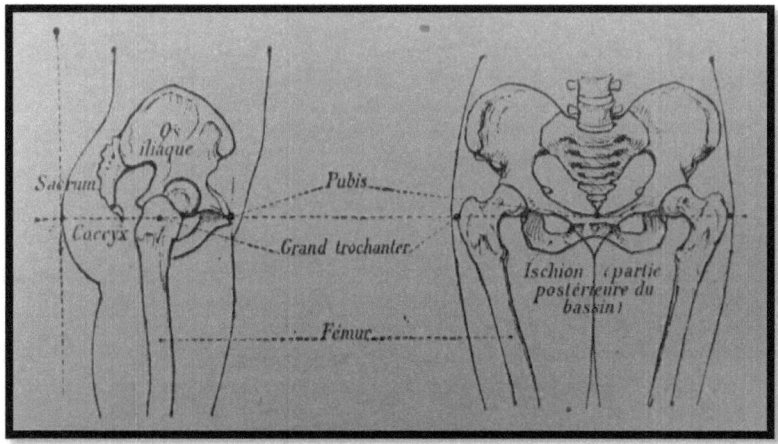

Figure 18. Plane of separation between the trunk and lower limbs. Depiction of the points determining this plane: upper edge of the pubis, external borders of the greater trochanter, tangential points with the vertical line of the buttocks.

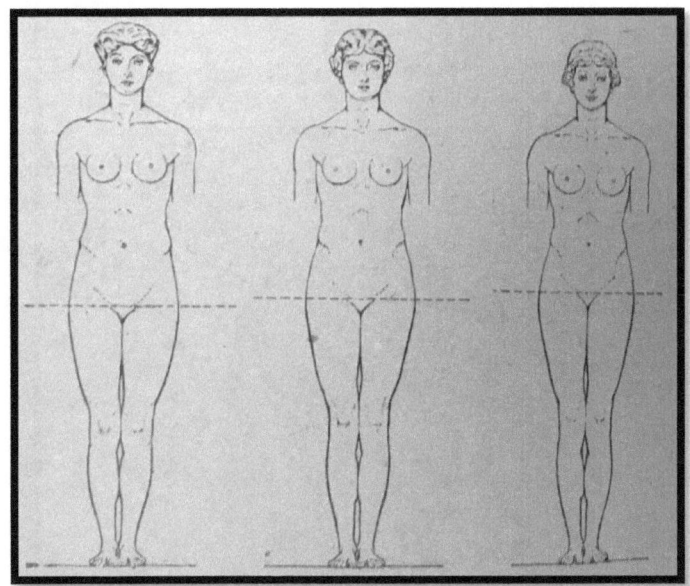

Figure 19. Trunk length and lower limbs comparison among three individuals having the same waist height. Center: the plane of separation of the trunk and lower limbs is the same as the middle of the body, proportions are normal. Left: the trunk and lower limbs separation is situated below the mid line of the body. The lower limbs are short and the trunk is long. Right: the plane of separation of the trunk and lower limbs is situated above the mid line of the body. The lower limbs are long and the trunk is short.

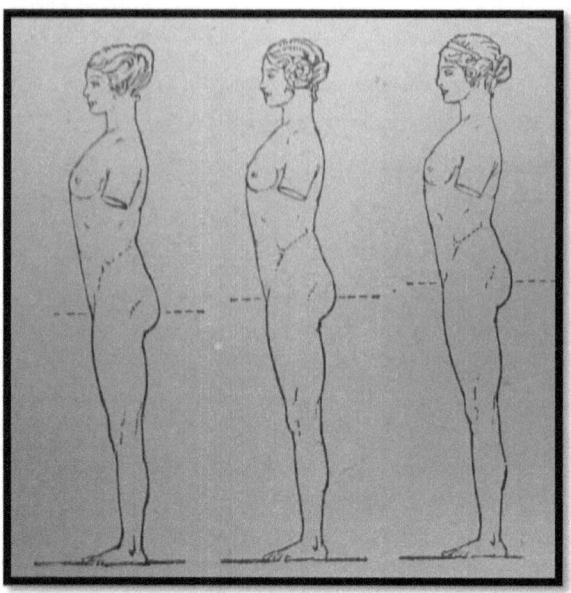

Figure 100. Trunk length and lower limbs comparison among three individuals having the same waist height Center: Normal proportions. Left: short lower limbs, long torso. Right: long lower limbs, short torso.

1) *Waist height.*

A woman can be beautiful with a nice build regardless of the waist height, so long as the proportions of the various body parts are in proper ratio to that height.

However, being too short, under 1.5m (about 5'), or too tall, above 1.85m (about 6'1"), constitutes a deviation only if the exaggeration of being too tall or too short becomes considerable.

The heights presenting the most advantages from the standpoint of practice of all kinds of exercises, which at the same time bring about the value of the elements of beauty are between 1.65m (5'4") and 1.75m (5'7 ½").

2) *Ratio of trunk to lower limbs. – Middle of the body.*

Standing, weight distributed on both legs straight and together, the middle of the body, which corresponds to half at waist height, is at or near the level of one of the following four points: lower extremity of the coccyx (tailbone), upper edge of the pubic bone, the external edge of the greater trochanters (hip bone) or the tangent point with a vertical line of the outer part of the buttocks.

Except in cases of bad build, these four points are generally at the same level, or with a small distance of one another (two centimeters at the most).

When the middle of the body is near these points, two centimeters above or below at the most, the trunk and leg proportions are regular.

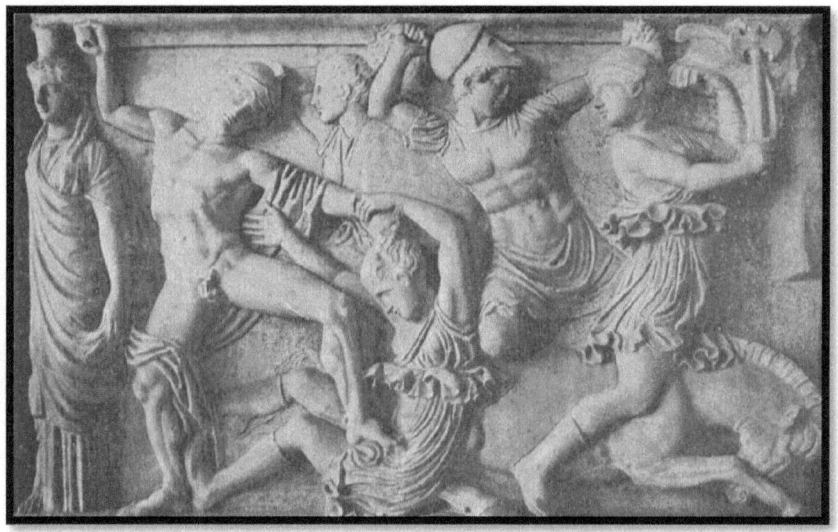

Sarcophagus depicting battles between Greeks and Amazons (Thessaloniki). Louvre museum, Paris.

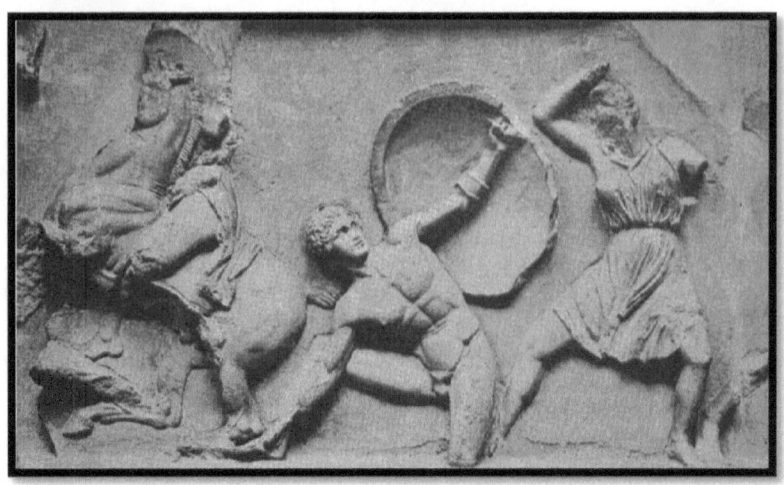

Amazons and Warriors (British museum, London)

Notice the superb deployment of the pectoral muscles of the kneeling warrior. These muscles constitute the beauty of the shape of the chest in men like in women.

### MUSCULAR DEFINITION IN MAN AND WOMAN

Male and female athletes with equally defined muscles.

At the peak of development and training, muscles are defined and their shape sharpens with more or less striated lines. Fat layers are either gone or insignificant.

When the middle of the body is two centimeters above these points, the lower limbs are short and the torso is long; if on the contrary it is two centimeters below, the lower limbs are long and the torso short, the distancing being more considerable.

Too short lower limbs constitute a deviation as much as too long lower limbs.

Women with a low basin or with short legs have a less graceful gait. When they sit, they can appear of average height, because of their long torso, but once standing they appear of short, stocky stature.

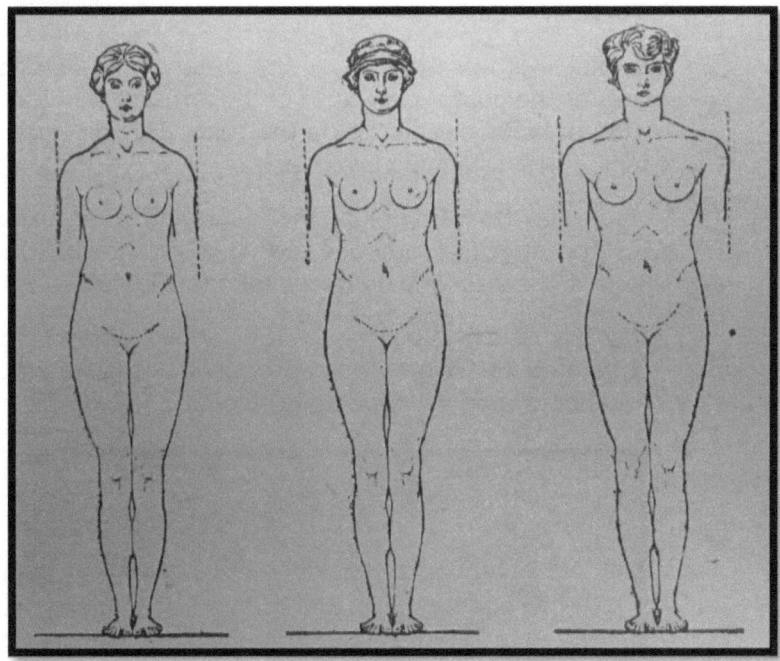

Figure 21. The build. Compared shoulder width in three individuals having the same height and basin thickness. Center: normal build. Left: weak build (gangly type). Right: strong build (masculine or stocky type).

The width of the basin influences the appearance of the lower limbs and gives a false sense of appreciation in regards to their length, when the waist height's center isn't checked in relation to the aforementioned four points.

For instance, narrow hips make the lower limbs appear long, whereas wide hips make them look shorter than they actually are.

Trunk and limb proportions tend to be incorrect when taking pictures, when the camera isn't positioned at the same level as the center of the waist height.

3) *Torso width or build.*

The total width of the torso is the distance, in a straight line, which separates the outermost edges of the arms (at shoulder height), when the upper limbs are alongside the body. This distance is quite easily obtained when standing in a doorway.

To align with the waist height, the torso width must be between 24 and 25% of the latter. For someone 1.65m tall (5'4"), the build varies between 0.396m at the least and 0.412m at the most (between 15 and 16 inches).

Below this ratio, the build is narrow; above, and it is too wide; when exaggerated, the narrow build produces this lanky type, called "wiry" or "beanpole", and the wide build stocky.

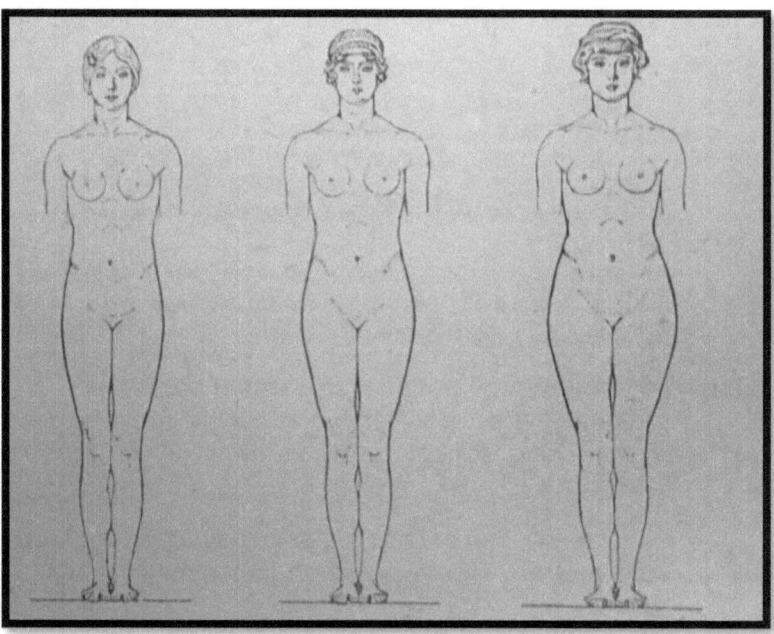

Figure 22. Hip width, comparison of the basin in three individuals having the same height and build. Center: normal width. Left: narrow width (gangly or masculine type). Right: wide hips (stocky type).

This build measurement comes from the width of the chest augmented by the muscular development of the shoulders. It can be also increased among people whose shoulder muscles are not fully developed, which is the case for most women.

4)   *Basin/hip width.*

The width of the basin is the distance in a straight line between the outermost edges of the hips. This distance is measured like that of the build, by standing in a doorway, the upper body leaning forward.

To be in harmony with the waist height and the torso width, the maximal width of the basin should be 20 to 21% of the waist height, so roughly 16% smaller than the maximal width of the shoulders' outermost points. For someone 5'4", this width is between 13 and 13.6 inches.

Lower, and the basin is too narrow; higher and it is too wide. Pushed to the extreme, narrowness produces a masculine type, while extreme width makes for a stocky build.

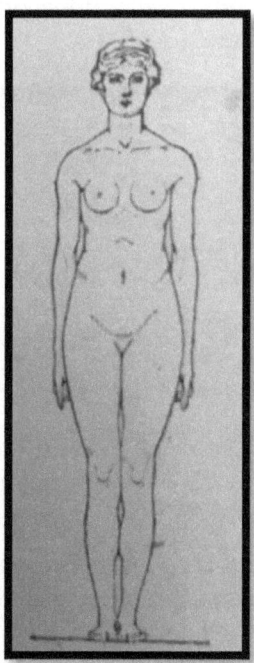

Figure 23. Bad attachment of the arms in relation to the hips. When the width of the hips is wider than normal or the build is too narrow, because of insufficient development, the arms cannot fall in place properly. Here the arms have to go back to stay in line with the shoulders

When the basin is too wide in relation to the shoulder build, the arms cannot fall in line with the shoulders and are obstructed by the hips. [PIX]

From there, there is a simple process to judge if the amplitude of the hips is normal.

The width of the basin in women is, at equal waist height, 10 to 15% greater than that of a man.

5)  *Chest thickness, from front to back – Anteroposterior thorax diameter.*

When the thorax conformation is regular, the breast line, from a profile view, starting at the neck, shows, when the upper body is upright, the back against a flat wall, an incline of about 45 degrees in relation to vertical alignment.

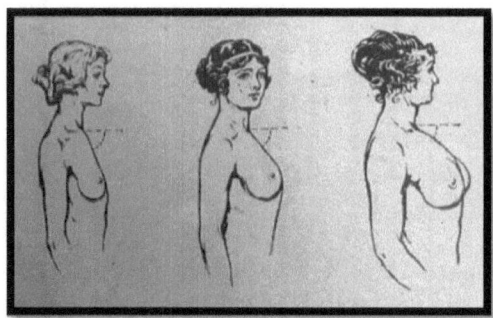

Figure 25. Thorax thickness. Center: normally open chest. The sternum line has an angle nearing 45º. Left: flat or caved in chest. Sternum nearly vertical. Right: thick chest. Sternum over-elevated.

The thickness od the chest is always good so long as this condition is met, regardless of the person's height. If the direction of the chest line is close to vertical, the thorax is flat; if it goes beyond the 45° angle, the thorax is too ample. In either case, the conformation is considered defective.

6) *Amplitude scale – Upper limbs length.*

This represents the distance between the extremity of the fingertips of the right hand to that of the fingertips of the left hand, the arms extended horizontally, with the back against a wall or the body flat on the ground (*wingspan*).

The wingspan thus gives us the length of the upper limbs, augmented by the width of the trunk; to be regular, it must be at least equal to the height or not exceed that measure by more than 2 cm (a little under 1 inch). If it exceeds it, it is considered long; if it doesn't reach at least the person's height, it is short.

When the upper limbs hang alongside the body, fully extended and shoulders low, the extremities of the extended fingers must fall close to mid-thigh level, or at the middle distance between the plane that separates the trunk from the lower limbs and the plane crossing the knees (line running below the patella), not to exceed that plane by more than 2 centimeters (under an inch).

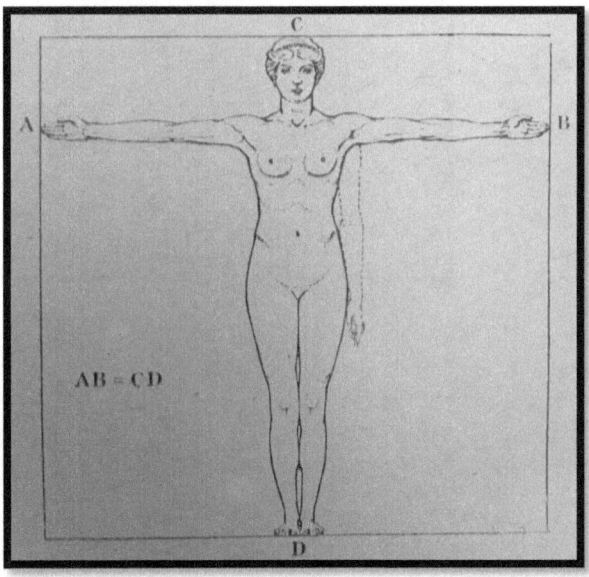

Figure 26. Wingspan, arms and fingers fully extended, in line wth the shoulders. This length is equal to the height of the individual, or exceeds it by about 2 cm at the most (under 1 inch).

When the fingertips do not reach at least mid-thigh level, the upper limbs are short; when on the contrary they exceed this distance by more than 2 centimeters, the upper limbs are long .

7)   *Knee position – Relative length of the thigh and the leg*

To determine the position of the knee, let us consider a plane running through the junction of the heads of the femur and the tibia, or, which comes out to about the same, the lower edge of the patella, or the knee pit.

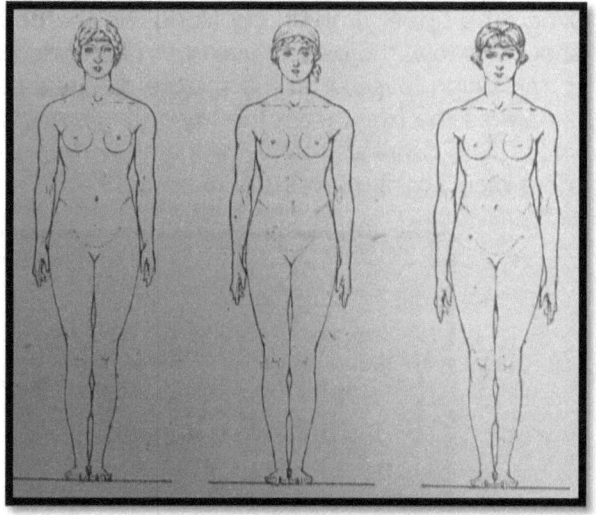

Figure 27. Comparing upper limbs length in three individuals having the same height and same plane in terms of trunk and legs separation. Center: normal length, fingertips at mid thigh, or half-distance between the plane separating the trunk from the lower limbs, that plane running across the hip bone. Left: arms too short. Right: arms too long.

For the knee to be properly positioned, the distance of this plane to the plane separating the trunk and the lower limbs (already described in the preceding point) must be greater than 1/10th to about 1/20th of the distance of the plane running through the internal edge of the ankle (at the tangential point of a vertical line with the internal malleolus or internal malleolus contact point when the legs are together). In other words, the knee (at the junction of the femur and the tibia) is not situated in the middle of the distance separating the upper part of the pubis of the internal malleolus of the ankle, it is slightly below. When the proportions are normal, the thigh is longer than the leg by about 5 to 10%, that distance being calculated on a vertical line when the body is standing.

When the distance of the knee to the separation of the trunk and the lower limbs doesn't reach 1/10 to 1/20 of the distance of the knee to the internal malleolus of the ankle, the thigh is short and the leg is long.

If the distance of the knee to the trunk separation line exceeds 1/10 to 1/20 of the distance of the knee to the malleolus, the thigh is long and the leg is short.

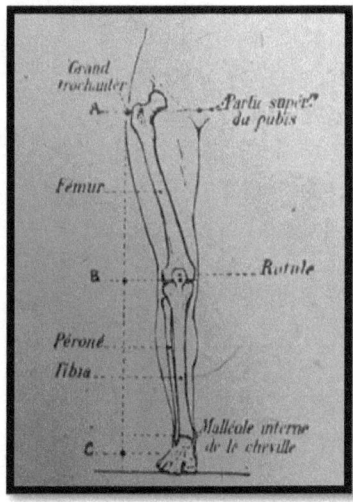

Figure 28. knee position. Comparing thigh and leg length. When the knee position is normal, the thigh is longer than the shin. The AB length is applied to the BC length, where C falls at the mid-point between the internal malleolus and the base of the foot. If C falls closer to the malleolus, the thigh is short and shin long. If on the other hand C falls closer to the base of the foot, the thigh is long and shin short.

Practically speaking, to obtain those measures, use a ruler or tape suffices, following the direction of a plumb line, when the body is standing, to calculate the distance of the upper part of the pubis to the junction of the femur and the tibia, which gives us the length of the thigh, and on the other hand, the distance separating the latter from the point of contact of the internal malleolus of the ankles when the legs are together, which gives us the length of the leg.

When the thigh has normal proportions, its length, noted with the ruler on the leg from the femur/tibia junction, falls more or less with the middle of the instep of the foot, between the internal malleolus and the foot's sole.

When the thigh is short, its observed length falls more or less close to the internal malleolus (below, sometimes above); when the thigh is long, on the contrary, this length comes close to the bottom of the foot.

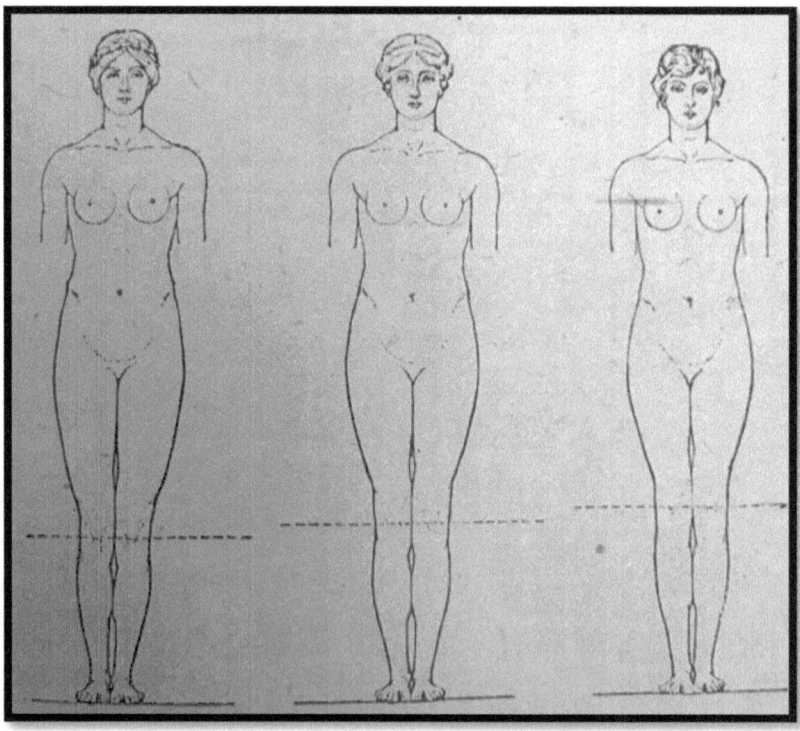

Figure 29. Comparative thigh and shin length among three individuals of the same height. Center: normal proportions. Left: short shin, long thigh. Right: long shin, short thigh.

A low knee, in humans, is the same as for animals and indicates that the lower limbs are more apt for running than jumping; a high knee indicates opposite aptitude, better for jumping than for running, not taking in consideration, in either case, the value of the musculature and vital organs, value which can modify greatly the results in both of these types of exercises.

A long thigh is a defect proportionally less frequent than a short thigh. The lower limbs with short thighs and longer calves, as some artists persist on drawing, a reminiscent of stilt-walking.

8) *Neck length*

The length or height of the neck isn't due only to the length of the cervical vertebrae comprised between the based of the skull and the first ribs. It rather depends on the degree of development of the trapezius muscles, which make up its posterior base, of the degree of lower or raising of the shoulders, of the position as well as the conformation of the upper maxillary, and finally to one's own size.

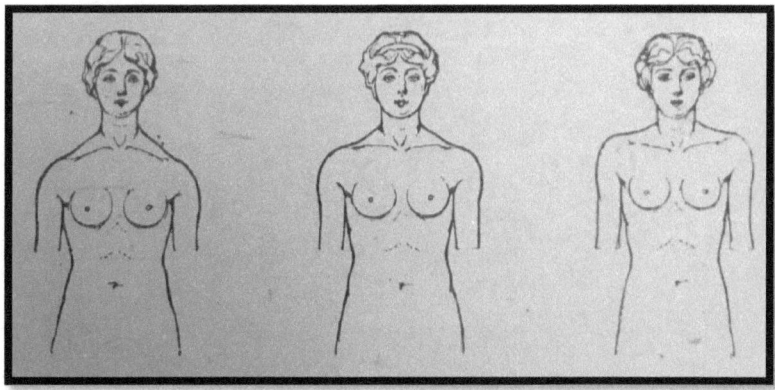

Figure 110. Shoulder height in three individuals of the same height (from maxillary to sternum) and same build. Center: normal shoulder position. Left: sloping shoulders. The neck seems long. Right: shrugged shoulders. The neck seems short.

Long or short looking necks are equally defective, more particularly both short and thick, or long and skinny on the contrary.

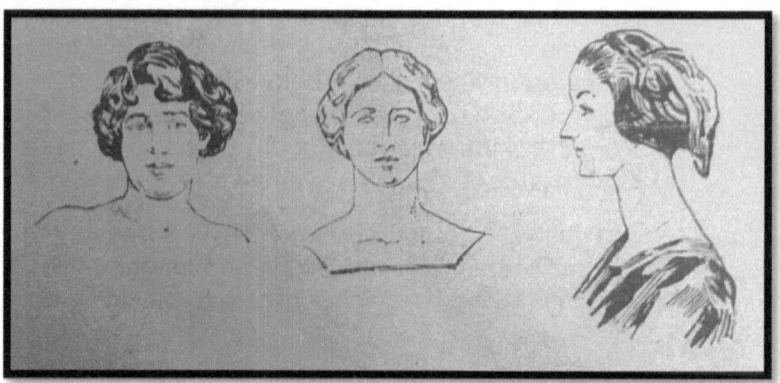

Figure 31. Comparative neck height. Center: normal height. Left: short neck or sunken into shoulders. Right: long neck, or "swan" neck.

When the shoulders are raised too much, the neck is called "dug into the shoulders"; when they are sloping and at the same time the lower maxillary is high, the neck is called "swan neck".

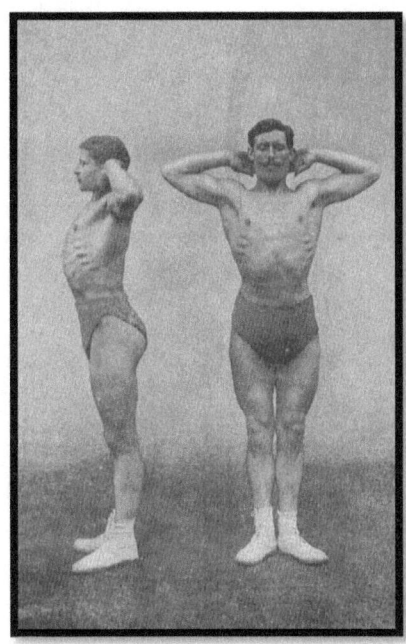 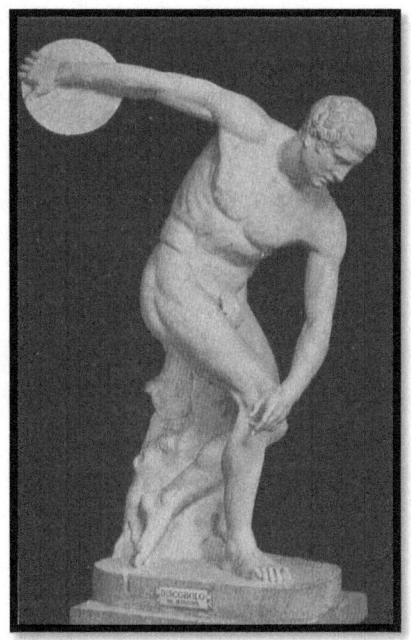

MUSCULAR DEFINITION IN MEN

Left: lean, natural types (author's students) in simple poses aiming to show muscular definition.

Right: Miron's Discus thrower (Vatican Museum)

Lean type with long muscles, whose contracted muscular segments are remarkably defined. Notice the shape of the pectorals, serratus, as well as the left calf.

9) *Feet and hands.*

It is difficult to precisely determine the dimensions of these two body parts. We admit generally to having the foot match the length of the forearm, from the tip of the elbow to the wrist bend, and that the hand must match the length of the face, from the chin to the upper edge of the forehead. But these points only refer to one dimension: length.

Exaggerations of size in either direction, too large or too small, are considered defective for either hands or feet.

Although too little is characteristic of weakness, it is however less disgraceful than too large.

10) *Thickness of joints: ankles, wrists, knees and elbows.*

Thick ankles, wrists, knees and elbows constitute a big defect.

The thickness of the bones in these areas proves a deformation caused by excess labor done by either the individual (farm work, domestic work...) or his or her ascendants; an exaggeration is size of the hands or feet comes from the same cause.

According to a well-spread opinion, fine ankles and wrists are a sign of purity or fineness in ethnic standards. It is correct. We will explain this with in details that the ideal type is the lean type, produced by the practice of natural exercises, whereas the stocky type with thick joints and big muscles is a deformity of the lean or natural types produced by the excess of strength work.

One must not confuse, however, being lean with being skinny due to being frail or with a weak bone structure, or some traces of childishness. An ankle, for instance, can be fine from an bone standpoint, but are still thick, especially when seen from the side, as a result of the power of the tendons attached to the leg muscles.

# CHAPTER IV : SHAPELY BEAUTY, OR MUSCULAR BEAUTY

## 23.  SHAPES. OUTLINE OR SILHOUETTE. CURVES. CONTOURED CURVES.

Shapes, as we already said, are made up of flesh. They depend mainly on the muscular development.

The exterior contour of the flesh determines *the line* or *silhouette*.

The general shape of the muscle will be described as *curves*.

The contours of the curves of the various muscles are drawn, especially during contractions, by actual lines, or even striation, more or less shaded or defined based on lighting.

The intersections of fascia in the same muscle, like the rectus abdominis for instance, are also show definition the same way.

The contours of the curves, just like the fascia line intersections, constitute important elements of the appreciation of shapes.

The sharpness of these lines is all the more perfected as the development of the muscles is achieved.

## 24.  VARIOUS ASPECTS OF MUSCULAR CURVES ACCORDING TO THE DEGREE OF DEVELOPMENT OR THE TRAINING CONDITION. MUSCULAR COVERING AND DEFINITION.

When a well-developed muscle becomes active, its curve sharpens dramatically.

The body isn't made up of permanently flat or smooth surfaces; it presents muscular projections more or less visible when at rest and quite pronounced when contracted.

The absence of projection (or level), flatness, or on the contrary the rounding of some areas, are proofs of an improper muscular development or accumulation of fatty tissue.

Several remarks are necessary to properly judge the value of muscular curves.

The curve/shape is more or less pronounced according to the degree of development or the current state of training. It is necessary to differentiate these two states, as one can have achieved integral development and find oneself, at any given moment, either in a non-active period or simple rest, or in a training period.

At the peak of development and at once during a training period, in other words in a "ready state", to use the expression used in sports, the shape of the muscles and the fascia lines are extremely sharp/defined.

The skin adheres to the muscle without fat in-between, or at least without a noticeable layer. Muscular fibers are even seen through the skin when the muscle is strongly flexed.

At the limits of extreme training, curves become "cut" and in the case of overtraining, remind a bit that of someone being "skinned". This applies to women as well as men.

When the training period ends, and it cannot last more than a few weeks or days without reaching overtraining, or as soon as normal activity slows, the muscles appear less "defined", small fat deposits fill in and soften the lines of external contours or the fascia. "Covering" takes place, more or less visible as the training load is reduced, compared to what it was prior, and a more abundant food intake. Flesh is then filled. [PIX]

This state of covering disappears easily in a few days or weeks as soon as training or regular activity resumes. If, by lack of exercise, we let that covering go on, we progressively suffer all the setbacks on health and beauty. Fattening begins.

We almost never see, in our civilized countries, except for a few circus professionals and sometimes dance professionals, female individuals with a degree of development or in a training state corresponding to the apex of development or training as seen in men. There aren't anymore Amazon women as there were during Antiquity.

All women, even the most actives ones or the athletic ones who play sports only for recreation and not to achieve the highest degree of development, have incompletely developed muscles that are always more or less covered with some fat. On the other hand, some fat deposits localized in specific areas of the body represent arthritic problems impossible to make go away completely, even through exercise.

It's this state of covering of the body, more or less pronounced, sometimes clearly overweight, that makes some say or believe, physiologists, doctors, artists and, in generally, almost all authors of dissertations on women's beauty, that in female subjects, rounded shapes, or in other words excess fat, is a normal shape.

Nothing is more incorrect and only proves the ignorance of the rearing of humans.

We confuse *what is*, as a result of the excessive covering or invasion of fat, a state caused solely by the insufficiency of physical exercise, with *what could be* and *should be*, if women were not in a habitual state of inactivity or physical laziness.

On another hand, it is important to note that, even outside of any excess fat, the state of insufficient muscular development shows in rounded shapes in certain areas, even if well developed in others. For instance, frail or atrophied limbs have an almost cylindrical shape.

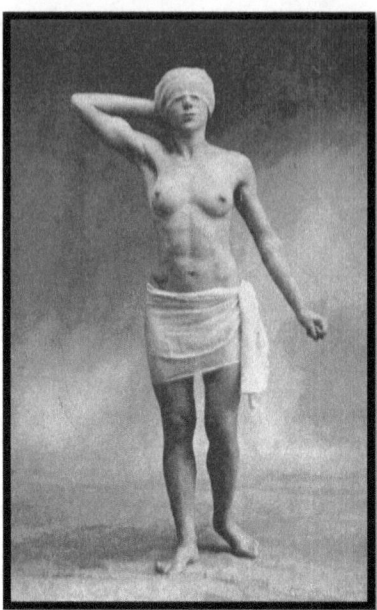 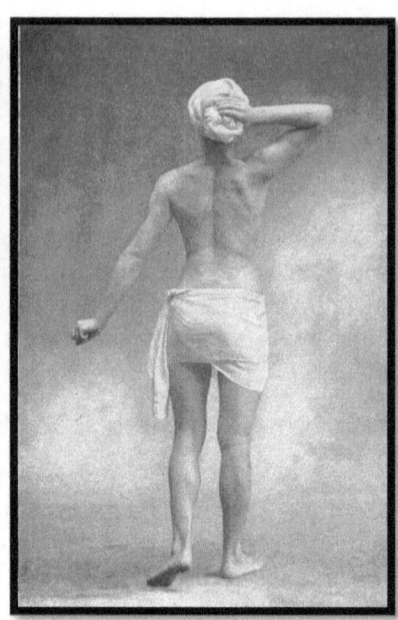

**MUSCULAR DEFINITION IN WOMEN**

Fully developed individual (author's student) in flexing poses to assess the level of muscular definition.

Left: pose showing the development of the shoulders, back and calves.

Right: pose showing the definition of the abdominal and oblique muscles, very sharp.

In skinny women, as well as overweight women, we can find the same shape defect: rounding.

The famous belief relative to rounded *feminine* curves is a cause of rejection by women towards muscle and sought by men. Such curves are not specific to women. Men whose physical life is also reduced, like that of some women, display rounded shapes either by excess fat, or by lack of development.

In primitive *active* cultures and races, developed women in training, "in shape" as goes the expression, have defined muscles as much as men in equal state of development or training. All those who witnessed indigenous women of exotic countries (porters, dancers, etc.), especially those belonging to warrior people, have immediately noticed this particularity.

The last Amazons, who disappeared at the same time as the last king of Dahomey, were, according to travelers, in impressive physical shape, identical to those of their most robust male companions.

In animal species, the same goes for females; there is no difference when compared to males. In horseracing, racing mare at their training peak display muscles just as clearly defined as the male horses. The covering appears in the mares as soon as training stops.

In summary, muscular *definition* is characteristic of the state of training or maximal activity; *simple covering*, average level of physical activity (maintenance), which is the normal state of training outside of maximal training intensity periods; *exaggerated covering,* a state of activity inferior or of weak training in relation to the vitality of the body (undertraining) and finally, *obvious overweight*, a state of complete inactivity or extremely weak, or also a specific state, which we will discuss, which has nothing to do with our natural needs. Nutrition also has an important role in the production of these various states.

Many women, quite busy or working a lot, to whom physical exercise is suggested for their well-being as well as their beauty, are quick to respond: "But I'm non-stop all day!" This proves that they do not grasp the difference between natural activity, which solely consists of the practice of natural and functional exercises, and all other types of activity that civilization imposed upon us.

By non-conforming activity to natural laws, we mean the execution of labors that can be extremely fatiguing (nervous fatigue, or localized in one area of the body...), which have nothing to do with natural exercises.

We can, for instance, rank in that category: all labors done by seamstresses, factory workers, typists, pianists, teachers etc.; work done by salespeople, cooks etc., work done kneeling (maids, etc.), and in general, all work done in a closed and restricted space. No work of such kind has any effect on the natural development, and most are, on the contrary, deforming.

Being too "cut", "dry" with a muscular definition reminiscent of a skinless body, when the muscles are at rest, is a defect just like excess fat is. However, while the latter is due to a lack of activity or excess inactivity, the "dryness" is on the contrary a result of the opposite excess: overtraining.

## 25. ALTERATION OF SHAPES CAUSED BY ADIPOSE TISSUE.

We know, anatomically speaking, that the body, in summary, is made up of bones, or the skeletal structure, internal organs, flesh or muscles, with skin covering it all. Except for a few very small surfaces, bones and internal organs are always covered by a more or less thick layer of muscle, whose shape the skin merely espouses.

But, outside of musculature, it is important to note the presence of adipose (fat) tissue spread here and there around the flesh and in various regions of the body. According to their importance of their level of thickness, these layers characterize one of the states we just defined: definition, simple covering, excess or exaggerated covering, and obvious overweight.

The thickness of fat layers is determined with a sufficient approximation using the following process, commonly used, and forgive us the analogy, by breeders, butchers or all animal handlers: one needs to pinch, between the thumb and index, or cupping with full hands in significant fat deposits, all the palpable tissue above the bones or muscles, and to measure the thickness of the roll thus formed.

When fat is absent, the roll in question is merely made up of twice the layer of skin, a thickness of about 1 to 2 millimeters between the thumb and index. We can baseline this minimal thickness by pinching the back of the hand of a skinny person.

Fat tissue is never uniformly spread on the surface of the body. It affects only certain parts. The specific areas are the following: the abdomen, flanks (from the belt to the shoulder blades), the low back, the chest and breasts, the armpits, the buttocks, the shoulders, the neck, the knees...

In a state of good definition, the fat layers are absent in some regions and insignificant in others. The thickness of the palpable roll above the bones or muscles is on average 2 or 3 millimeters and barely exceeds ½ centimeter in specific regions of deposits that we just mentioned. The curves of the muscles when contracted are pure and intact.

In a simple state of development, the thickness of the palpable roll is on average 3 to 5mm and barely exceeds 1cm in the aforementioned areas.

Among fully developed individuals, simple covering is not a defect. It is a natural consequence of the stopping of higher intensity training or maximal activity. Fat layers only slightly soften muscular definition.

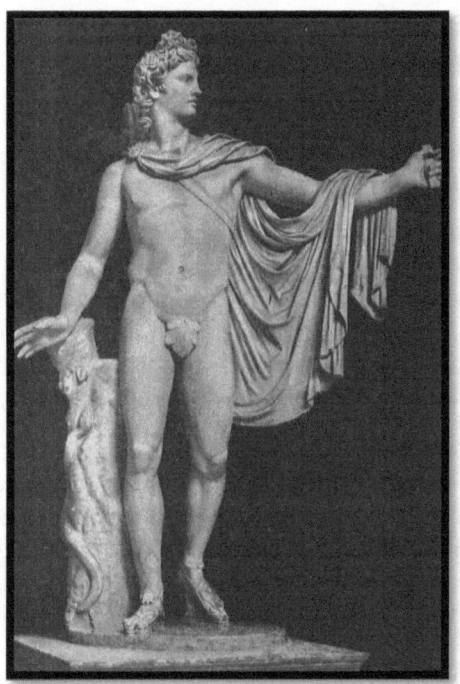 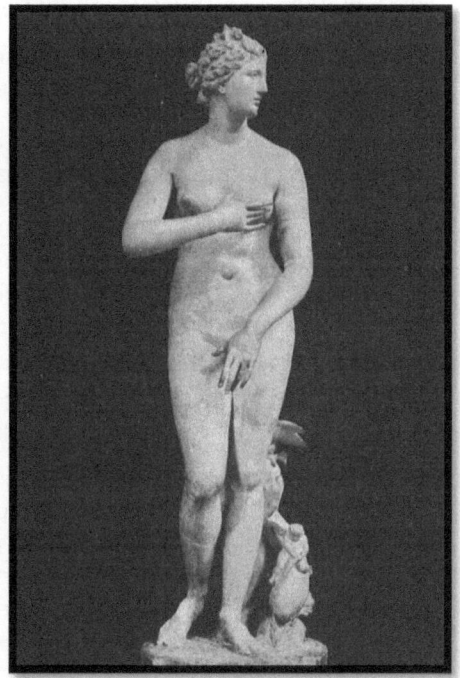

"COVERING" OF THE SHAPES IN MEN AND WOMEN

*Left: Belvedere's Apollo* (Vatican museum).

*Right: Medici's Venus* (Florence)

The simple covering is characteristic of a thin layer of fat, which covers the muscles, removing some definition, and tends to soften the shape. Simple covering is a normal state among developed individuals, outside of intense training periods.

Beyond 2cm of thickness, the overweight condition begins. It is slight between 2 and 3cm, average between 3 and 4cm, strong between 4 and 5cm, and finally very strong above that limit.

Adiposity (storage of fat) constitutes a concern from an esthetic standpoint. Fat deposits hide the definition of the muscles, modify the curves and consequently alter shapes and destroy it. They fill in the normal depressions or dips: armpits, sternal notch, elbow and knee pits, etc. They form rolls and abnormal folds, mainly at the flanks, buttocks etc.; they make the limbs appear rounded. Finally, they produce a swelling of the face, a generally stocky appearance and make the body look heavy.

Obesity, which is nothing but strong or extreme adiposity, is at the upper limit of ugliness, when it doesn't become monstrous.

A fat person, or adipose, even if a little bit, average or strongly, is considered unattractive, as their shapes are no longer normal.

Outside of this setback affecting beauty, adiposity indicates a body in inferior health condition, overloaded with useless or hazardous elements, liable to cause a morbid condition at any given moment. A current notion considers it both a reserve of health or a proof of vitality. The simple rotundness that some doctors have even gone so far as to recommend, and to which many indulgences have been allowed, is nothing but light or moderate adiposity.

When the fat layers are reduced to a minimum, as seen in clear muscular definition or normal covering, their weight should range, according to some anatomists, between 5 and 1015 max of the total body weight (thus 3 to 6kg - 6.5 to 13lb- for a person weighing 60kg/132lb). In the cases of obesity, it can reach 25%. An overweight person weighing 80kg/176lb of total body, for instance, could be carrying an overload of about 20kg/44lb of fat.

Overweight persons are a byproduct of civilized life. There is no obesity, not even a little excess fat, in any primitive people leading a naturally *active* life, not any more than among free-living animals. Only some domesticated and inactive, gluttonous animals display traces of obesity.

As a result of a complete aberration of any esthetic sense, some oriental cultures consider an overweight, even obese state, as a state of beauty in women, inasmuch as they are kept away from any physical effort.

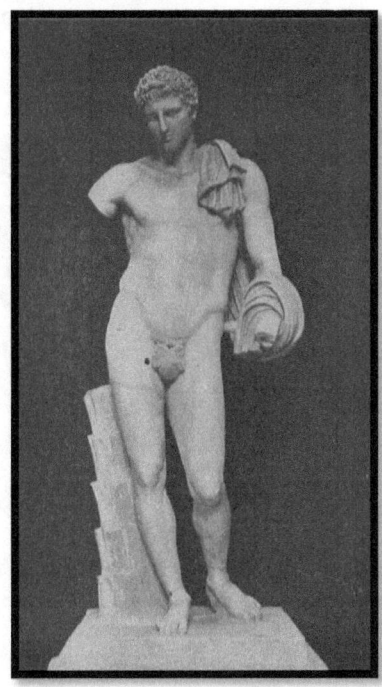 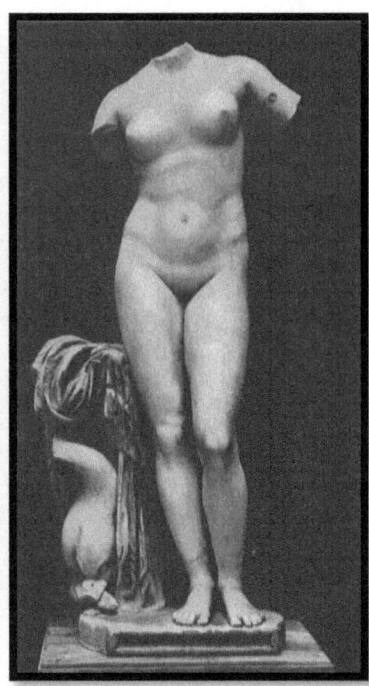

COMPARATIVE STUDY OF THE WAISTLINE AND THE SHAPE OF THE ABDOMEN IN MEN AND WOMEN.

Left: Antinoüs (Belvedere's Mercury) (Vatican museum, Rome).

Athlete with good definition. This pose allows comparing the similarity between the lateral line of the waist between this and the photo of Venus next to it. Also to compare the shape and lines of the lower limbs.

Right: Venus Anadyomene (Rome)

Here, the abdominal muscles are not as clearly defined as on the athlete's on the left, as it depicts with "covering". However, the abdominal line, the shape of the obliques and the stomach are still clearly visible and can be compared to the Antinoüs.

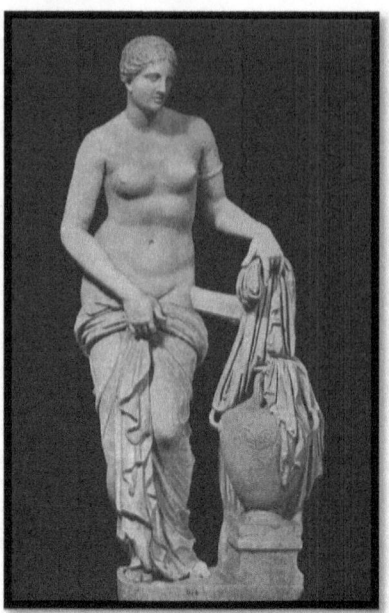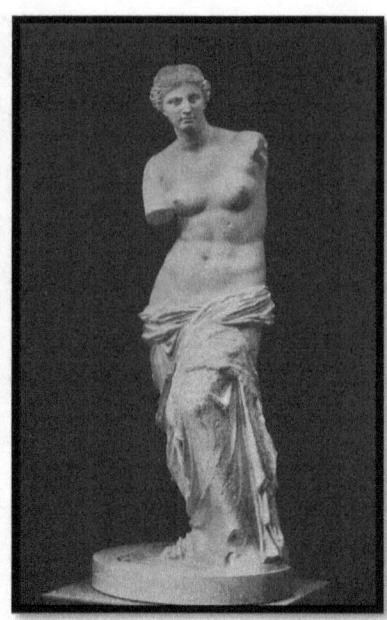

STUDY OF THE SHAPE OF THE ABDOMEN

NATURAL WAIST

Left: Cnidus's Venus (Vatican museum, Rome).

Notice the waistline, the shape of the rectus abdominis, the muscular roundness of the lower stomach, and the pectoral definition near the armpit, on which the breast is strongly attached.

Right: Venus of Milo (Louvre museum, Paris).

Notice the development of the abdominals, whose two transverse muscular lines are visible, as well as the lower stomach and the pectoral development.

# 26. DISTINCTIONS TO ESTABLISH BETWEEN MUSCULAR CURVES. THIN MUSCLES AND ROPY MUSCLES. LEAN OR NATURAL TYPE. MASSIVE TYPE AND INTERMEDIARY TYPE.

The same muscle doesn't have the exact same shape in all individuals. It can display under two opposite aspects: lean or knotty.

In women like in men, a normally shaped muscle, pure or natural, is a long, svelte and supple muscle.

A thick, short and knotty muscle is nothing more than an alteration of the lithe or natural muscle with excess strength training.

The differences in appearance indicated above are mostly characteristic in the limbs.

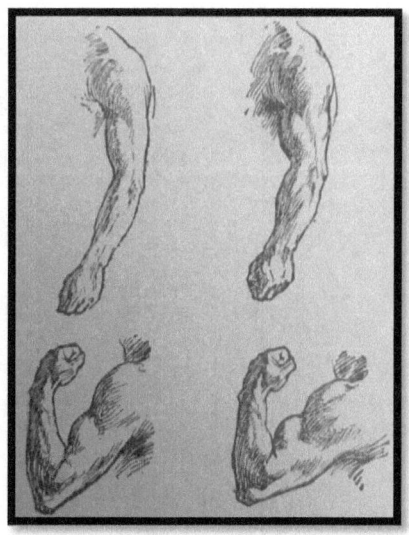

Figure 32. Lean, long muscles (natural) and short, knotty muscles (altered). This comparison of two types of muscles of the upper body shows them in a rested state as well as contracted. Left: natural. Right: altered. At rest, the shape of the lean muscle is barely noticeable, by contrast to the altered, overdeveloped larger muscle. Lean muscles only show a pronounced shaped when flexed. A noticeable difference in size/thickness exists between a relaxed versus a flexed muscle. The bigger muscles show their definition at rest as well as during contraction, and the difference in thickness between relaxation and contraction is barely noticeable.

At rest, the lithe or natural muscle shows little curve; its contour is barely noticeable. At the touch, it is relatively soft and of remarkable suppleness.

As soon as it is contracted, its curve juts out all the more strongly as its development is complete and the level of general fitness is high. At the touch, it then becomes extremely hard.

The thick, short and knotty muscle, on the contrary, seems constantly contracted, even at rest. It remains always hard to the touch and at the moment it gets activated, its curve changes very little. It is nearly as massive at rest as contracted, whereas a noticeable difference, in thickness or in shape, always exists between rest and contraction in the natural muscle.

A natural muscle gives the body as a whole a lean appearance; the thick or massive muscle has a heavy appearance. From here come out two opposite types: the lean and the massive.

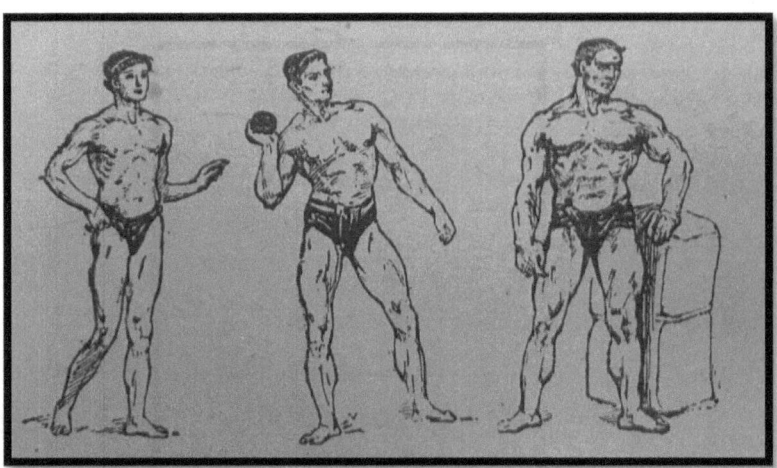

Figure 33. Lean, natural type and its alterations. The three types of muscular development, produced by three different approaches to train. Left: lean, thin or natural type (compared to the race horse). Center: medium type, semi-thin, semi-massive (light duty pulling horse). Right: massive or Herculean type (heavy labor pulling horse). The medium and massive types represent alterations of the thin type. They result from training where pure strength exercises dominate over speed and displacement drills.

Between these two extreme types, there is a class categorized of various average, or intermediary, semi-lean or semi-massive types, more or less close or distant from the characteristics of one or of the other.

Genetics contribute greatly to the development of these various body types, the lean, the median, the heavy; but the type of exercises or work practiced routinely during childhood and adolescence also has a strong influence on muscular development in one direction or another.

Natural and functional exercises, when displacement exercises dominate, produce a lean type, thus defined as pure and natural. With regular proportions, this is the ideal type of beauty.

Strength training (carries, farm work..), exercises of pure muscular development (apparatus gymnastics, weights, barbells…), simple muscular development equipment (cables, bands…) produce a massive type.

Finally, strength training exercises, alleviated by the practice of displacement exercises (running, walking, jogging), produce a medium type.

A powerful example of these different types can be provided to us in the animal kingdom with equine species.

The racehorse, or thoroughbred, light horse, lithe and svelte, elegant and supple; the draft horse or slow strength, big, short, massive and heavy; and the ponies, for pulling or light duty, semi-lean, are the products of three different types of training.

Dogs that are made to pull sleds, for instance, tend to take on a more massive shape, or medium, just like horses.

The lean type, as we said, is the pure or natural type. The massive or medium types close to the massive type are the former natural type, transformed or more accurately formed by the exclusive or exaggerated practice of exercises or labors of force/strength.

The human being, much like the animal, loses shape when it stops displacement training, or speed training, to turn into a draft or pulling horse.

Arabic cultures consider a horse to have lost its purity, its finesse, in one word its beauty, when it has been used as a draft horse. It's a setback without remedy; it is rejected as a breeding stallion. The racehorse is, indeed, the natural type of the equine species.

Several generations are usually needed to modify the type and determine the specific characteristics in shapes as well as proportions. However, the lean type is easily transformed, either into a medium or heavy type, if specializing in training or labors of strength, especially in slow labors, without any speedy movements of the body.

As for the massive type acquired via genetics, it is not possible to bring to a lean type. We can only modify to an extent.

Ignoring the development of these body types produces misunderstandings and is the primary cause of preconceived notions when it comes to muscular development.

Many women think that when partaking in exercising, they will develop an extreme massive type. To that, they have several excuses. They can, indeed, be struck by the sight of these Herculean bodies, with poor proportions, which some publications or some authors persist in displaying like models of beauty and strength. Then, at the sight of some of their peers practicing sports but who, by genetics, have inherited a medium or massive type, remain more or less massive, sometime even increasing their size or shape with improperly chosen exercises.

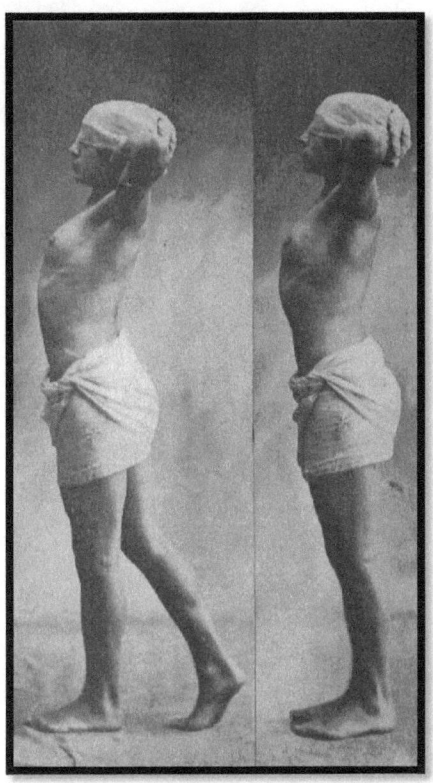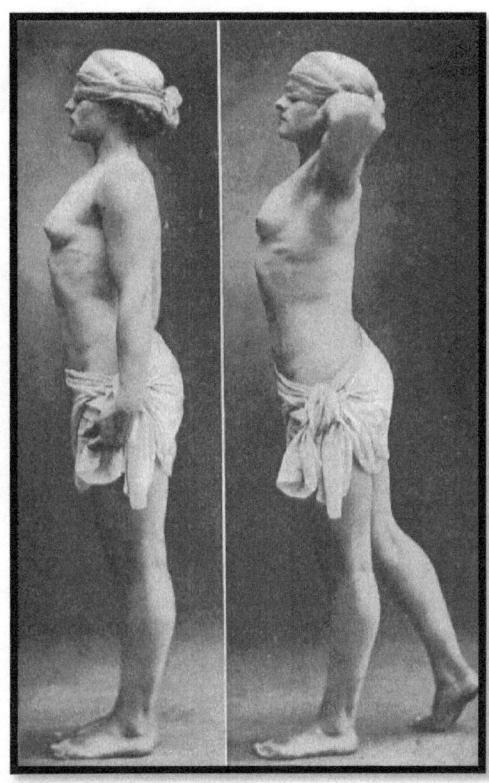

STUDY OF THE SHAPE OF THE ABDOMEN

Normal shape of the stomach line, profile view, in two fully developed individuals (author's students)

In the left two poses: normal shape of the stomach line mid-inhale or mid-exhale. From the tip of the sternum to the pubis, the line is straight or nearly straight.

In the right two poses: normal line at the end of an inhale or exhale. The stomach is slightly hollowed. Notice also the development of the serratus in both individuals.

Finally, at the example of some of their friends who have acquired short and thick muscles who trusted the development of their bodies to ignorant people, charlatans of physical culture, or simply by the sole use of strength training equipment: cables, dumbbells...

We understand that nothing more is needed to spread doubt and hesitation in their minds.

Let us reiterate that the natural method, faithful image of training and living naturally, will not bring this about, as it leads only to the development of the lithe and svelte type, which is once again, the natural type for beauty.

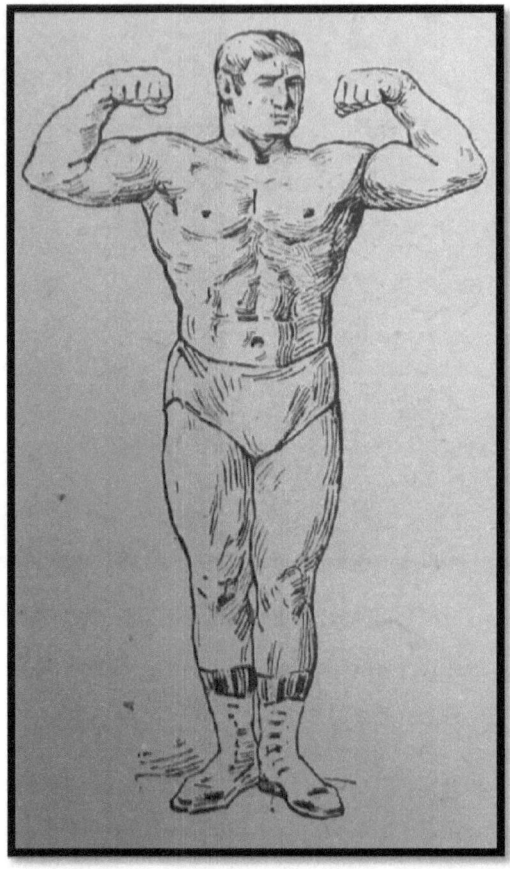

Figure 34. Herculean type of wrestler or weight lifter, presented to crowds as an ideal of strength and beauty.

# 27. ANTIQUE SHAPES

The following observation has never been made by authors of beauty treaties, at least not by anyone known to us. This proves once again that those who believe in rounded or fatty shapes as being the normal shape of a woman.

Let's refer to Antiquity statues. The artists of the time, quite keen on physical culture, have presented us with proper athletes, with muscular definition, indicative of a superior level of training.

Following the nature of these athletes and the type of exercises they would practice, the sculptors would either show a svelte type, with lean and long muscles, or a massive type, with short and thick muscles, or intermediate types having characteristics of one or the other of the former types.

When not displaying athletes, artists of Antiquity took care to show individuals with at least slight development. The statues of Apollo, Bacchus, etc. are strong examples of this difference in appearance. This is what led many authors to assign Apollo, for instance, effeminate curves! Apollo is simply "covered", because of not being in training condition the way athletes were. But that doesn't prevent him from being remarkably muscularly developed.

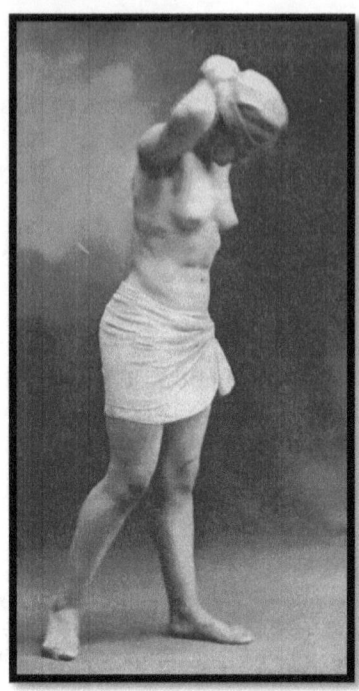 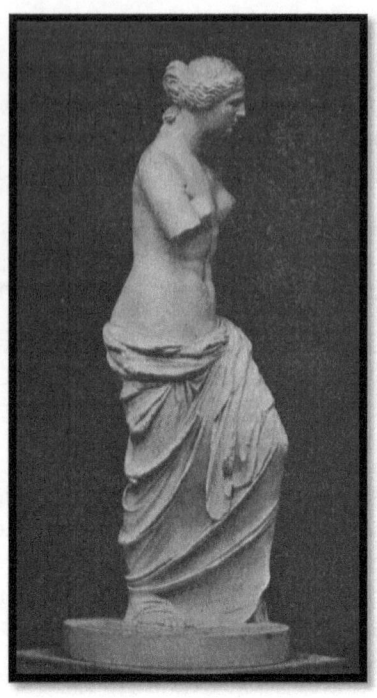

STUDY OF THE SHAPES OF THE ABDOMEN

Similarity of the muscle shape of the abdominals on the Venus of Milo and a young female athlete (author's student). Similarity of the low back line.

In order to be able to see her stomach, the young athlete raised her arm. Despite the fact that this position makes moving difficult, she replicates a muscular look identical to that of her renowned "rival".

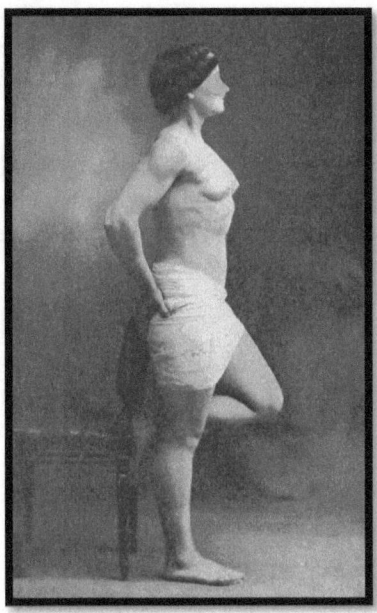 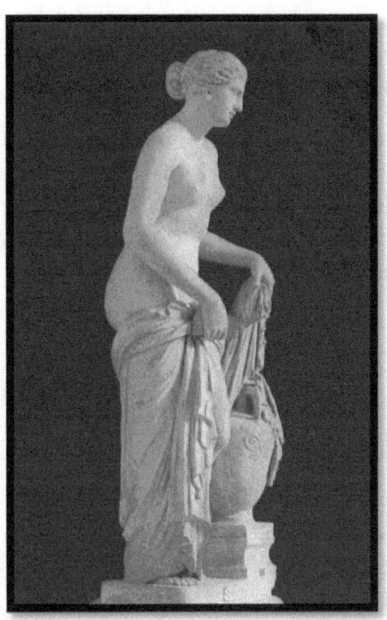

COMPARATIVE STUDY OF THE ABDOMEN'S SHAPES ON A STATUE FROM ANTIQUITY (Cnidus's Venus) AND A YOUNG FEMALE ATHLETE (Author's student).

Notice the nearly identical abdominal line (slightly hollowed, as normal towards the end of an inhale or an exhale) as well as of the low back line.

The arm of the Venus is at rest, whereas the right arm of the athlete shows contracted muscles, which explains the difference in shape of the arms.

Regarding statues representing women, what do we see? Here as well, the artist of that era paid attention to establish a difference between the untrained woman and the trained woman.

The untrained woman is always in a simple state of "covering". For example: any statue of Venus, whose muscular curves are simply softened in definition. But none is ever incompletely muscular or overweight.

As for the trained woman, the athletic woman, she possesses muscles as defined as a man's. Examples: all the Diane statues, the Spartan Runner and especially Amazons, which represent the ideal prototype of integral development.

Finally, as for men, the Antiquity artist distinguishes the lean and lithe woman's type, the average or intermediate type, and the massive type, depending on the case or the "ideal" to represent.

This short incursion into the works of art from the Antiquity era confirms what we already claimed on the subject of the identity of muscular development in both men and women. The appearance of this development varies, in either gender, according to the level of activity and the type of exercises routinely practiced.

## 28. HARMONY OF MUSCULAR DEVELOPMENT. MEASUREMENTS OF THE LIMBS AND THE TRUNK.

In order to be in harmony with the proportions and the height of the body, muscular development must satisfy certain conditions of width or thickness.

It is evident that, for instance, the lower limbs not be too frail with upper limbs too thick by contrast; the look would be lacking grace and esthetics.

It is as a result interesting to know the value of normal or regular measurements of the limbs and the trunk according to various heights.

The following numbers are given according to height and are characteristic of the lean or natural type.

Measurements of a value inferior to normal measurements characterize types with insufficient muscular development, skinny or even frail.

Measurements of a value superior to normal measurements characterize on the contrary the types with massive shapes, stocky or overweight.

In either of the last two cases, imbalances of weakness or excessive mass are all the more considerable as they are farther away from the norm.

The measurements of the various body parts are taken with a measuring tape directly applied to the skin, without squeezing forcibly. It is necessary to take several measurements at the same spot to reduce errors as much as possible.

1) *Chest.*

The chest circumference doesn't only depend on the amplitude of the thoracic cage, but also on the development of the dorsal (back) muscles, trapezius muscles and pectoral muscles.

This circumference measurement is obtained by placing the tape under the arms, hanging, under the armpits and right above the upper contour of the breasts. The tape, thus positioned, is not in a horizontal plane, rather slightly inclined. The measurement is calculated with both a powerful inhale and exhale. The two numbers must fall between 52 and 56% of the individual's height.

Example: for a height of 1.65m (5'4"), the chest circumference should have measurements falling between 0.858 at the low end and 0.924m on the high end (respectively about 34" and 36.5"). The following measurements of 0.88m (34.5") upon exhale and 0.91m (36") upon inhale are thus quite standard.

2) *Waist or belt.*

The waist circumference measurement is obtained by placing the tape at the narrowest spot. It must fall between 38 and 40% of the person's height.

Example: For a height of 1.65m (5'4"), the waist circumference ought to fall between 0.627m (25") and 0.66m (26").

3) *Neck.*

The neck measurement is obtained by placing the tape at the narrowest spot, which is found at about mid-neck height. This measure ought to fall between 20 and 21.5% of the height.

Example: For a height of 1.65m (5'4"), the neck circumference ought to fall between 0.33m (13") and 0.354m (14").

4) *Straight arm and flexed arm.*

These straight arm measurement and that of the flexed arm (biceps maximally contracted) is obtained by placing the tape around the thickest part, at about mid-biceps.

For the straight arm, the measurement ought to fall between 18 and 19%, and for the flexed arm between 20 and 21.5% of the height.

Example: For a height of 1.65m (5'4"), the width of the straight arm can vary between 0.297m (11.5") and 0.313m (12.33"), and that of the flexed arm between 0.33m (13") and 0.354m (14").

5) *Forearms.*

The circumference measurement of the forearm is obtained by placing the tape on the thickest part. It ought to fall between 14 and 15% of the height.

Example: For a height of 1.65m (5'4"), it can vary between 0.231m (9.1") and 0.247m (9.7").

6) *Thighs.*

The thigh circumference measurement is obtained by placing the tape on the thickest portion, right below the start of the buttocks. It ought to fall between 31 and 33% of the height.

Example: For a height of 1.65m (5'4"), it can vary between 0.51m (20") and 0.544m (21.4").

7) *Calves.*

The calf circumference measurement is obtained by placing the tape on the thickest portion. It ought to fall between 20 and 21.5% of the height.

Example: For a height of 1.65m (5'4"), the calf circumference ought to fall between 0.33m (13") and 0.354m (14").

It is important to note that the measurements of the calf, neck and flexed arm are very close to one another. All three fall, indeed, between 20 and 21.5% of the height.

Generally speaking, the calf is slightly thicker, whereas the flexed arm (biceps contracted) is slightly thinner than the neck; or, if preferred, the decreasing order of thickness of these three body parts is the following: calf, neck, flexed arm. However, it can happen that all three measurements are equal.

We have made a note on several occasions in the previous chapters that some individuals, while possessing only an under-developed musculature, could, however, when clothed, present a normal aspect ratio, thanks to well-distributed fat tissue. We now understand how this could be so: the thickness of the fat layers can be such that the measurements fall within the limits established above.

# CHAPTER V : THE ABDOMEN AND ITS DEFORMITIES

## 29. THE ABDOMINAL BELT. ITS LINE AND NORMAL CURVATURE.

The abdomen extends from the bottom of the ribs all the way to the basin. In this area, no skeletal structure support the layer of muscles that solely holds and protects major vital organs such as the stomach, the liver, the intestines, etc....

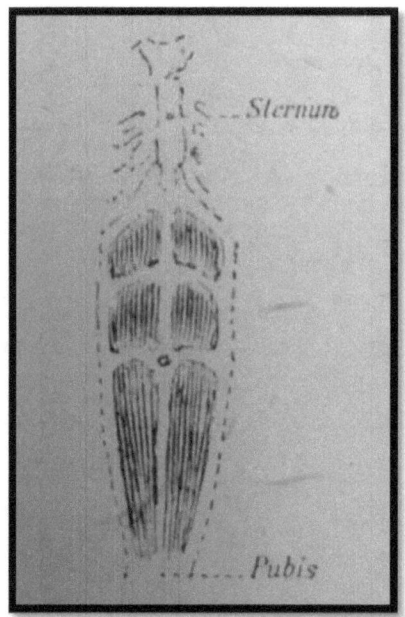

Figure 35. The abdominal wall. The rectus abdominis, their attachment points on the ribs and pubic bone, their six main myofascial intersections (three horizontal and three vertical) and their two muscular "bumps/rolls" above the navel.

The superficial musculature of the abdomen is made up of two groups of muscles: the *rectus abdominis* (*the 6-pack, "straight abs"*) and the *obliques*, whose development constitutes the beauty of the belly as well as that of the waist.

To be able to discover the lack of development or changes in shape of any belly/stomach, it is necessary to be knowledgeable in the normal shape of these muscles. A study from an esthetic standpoint, not just from an anatomical standpoint of the abdominal belt, is needed for that. It can easily be done on an Antique nude.

The *straight abs* are two symmetrical muscles in relation to the centerline of the body; they extend from the tip of the sternum and the cartilage of the nearby ribs all the way to the pubis. They form two elongated bands of muscles, separated by a median groove, which extends anatomically from the tip of the sternum to the navel, as well as the pubis, but is apparent on the naked boy only to the navel. In the upper section of the abdomen, a slight groove, visible on the naked body, marks the lateral contours of each of these muscles.

This groove is situated more or less at a like distance of the median groove to the lateral edges of the body.

These three grooves are nearly parallel and consequently vertical when the naked body is in an upright stance.

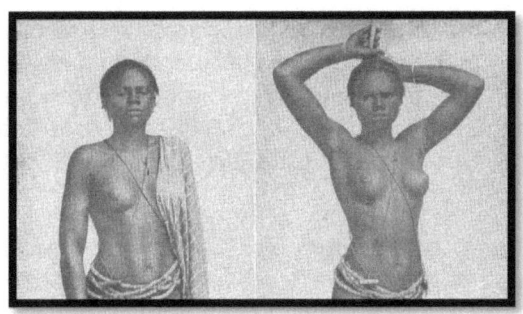 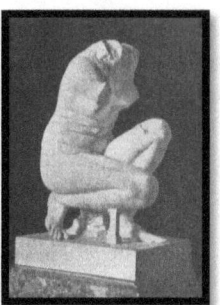

STUDY OF THE SHAPE OF THE TORSO AND UPPER LIMBS ON A PRIMITIVE TRIBAL WOMAN (TWO LEFT PHOTOS)

Note the shape of the arms whose definition appears when contracted, as well as the development of her abdominal muscles, especially the two vertical lines of the rectus abdominis, clearly visible, the firmness of her breasts attached to the pectoral muscles, compare to the previously shown photographs of Amazon warriors.

STUDY OF THE SHAPES OF THE ABDOMEN (FAR RIGHT)

Kneeling Venus (Louvre museum, Paris)

Notice the two transverse rolls of muscle of the abdominals.

From sternum to navel, the straight abs, instead of making up a continuous mass of flesh, or being one piece, are divided into two parts, connected by narrow fascia. As a result of this particular conformation, when the straight abs (rectus abdominis) contract, they fold like an accordion, and form two muscular rolls, superimposed across the stomach instead of producing a jutting muscle like a biceps would, for instance.

These two rolls, about the same in volume, are always apparent when contracted. The upper roll, smaller, is usually less pronounced than the lower.

Three sinuous transverse lines, at the end of some light grooves, draw up the contours of the two rolls. The lowest line comes close to the navel; the highest line is just below the sternum; the third, or median, the most pronounced, holds the middle between the other two.

The shape of the straight abs is thus formed of six lines, of which the first three, going lengthwise vertically with the body, form its junction as well as the lateral contours, and the other three, in a transverse direction, draw the edges or fascia intersection of the fleshy muscles. These six lines are perfectly visible, in their entirety or partially, even if the muscle isn't contracted, with "defined" individuals or with simple covering.

On the *Venus of Milo*, whose abdominal muscles are contracted, the two rolls of muscles are very sharp and the median transverse line is more defined than the others.

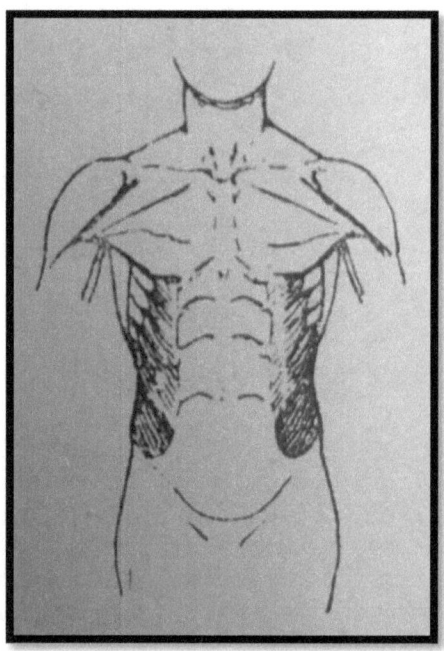

Figure 35. The abdominal wall and oblique muscles

In contraction, the straight abs, which are very powerful muscles, offer a remarkable hardness. They can, in that state, sustain a great blow, like a punch or an elbow strike, without much setback.

The straight abs get activated in just about any kind of effort, be it pulling, pushing, supporting, jumping, climbing, etc. Their shape is especially visible when one pulls or pushes an object placed ahead of the body, or, when hanging by the hands, one lifts the legs up, or, lying on the back, performing a sit-up.

The *oblique muscles* fill the lateral area of the abdomen, from the bottom of the ribs to the back of the iliac crest and the pubis.

Their development constitutes the beauty of the belt, specifically, and determines the waistline. Their external contour indeed forms a lateral bodyline, front or side, from bottom of ribs to hips.

During contraction, the trunk flexed laterally for instance, or simply in upright stance with the weight of the body on one leg, they appear as squared mass of muscles right above the hip bones.

In men, this build-up of muscles spills beyond the hip bones, but in women, the width of the basin softens this appearance, which exists nevertheless.

The oblique muscles get engaged in twisting or lateral flexing of the body, which happens especially in throwing exercises, single-leg balancing exercises, etc.

Generally speaking, just like the straight abs, they work more or less in all types of muscular efforts.

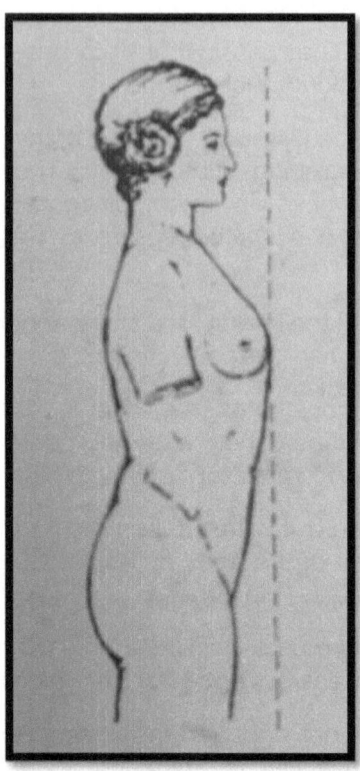

Figure 37. Normal shape of the abdominal line at mid-inhale or mid-exhale. To better appreciate the abdominal line, the trunk is upright, chest open, stomach inside a vertical line drawn from the tip of the sternum, the neck straight. This line isn't set. Its angle varies depending on the amplitude of the breathing movements. It is nearly vertical during mid-inhales or mid-exhales.

To finish, it is important to indicate the shape that the line of the stomach presents, when seen from the side. Imagine the body upright and with a correct posture, like when one is back to a wall, from heels to head. In this position, the line of the stomach, from a profile view, only display sight curves (when breathing normally), close to a straight line, which would join the pubis to the tip of the sternum. When inhaling or exhaling forcefully, the curves (convex or concave) become more pronounced between the sternum and the navel.

At the mid-point of the inhale or the exhale, we could say that the stomach line is nearly straight. However, such a look exists only among individuals possessing a perfect abdominal musculature, fully developed, in a superior state of training or conditioning.

It is nearly impossible to find, among modern civilized women, a stomach with an impeccable line, as a result of lack of physical activity and the continuous wear of corsets. It is important to note that it's only in the correct upright stance that the line of the stomach displays the above description. As soon as the trunk leans forward, muscular rolls protrude and clearly change the shape of the line.

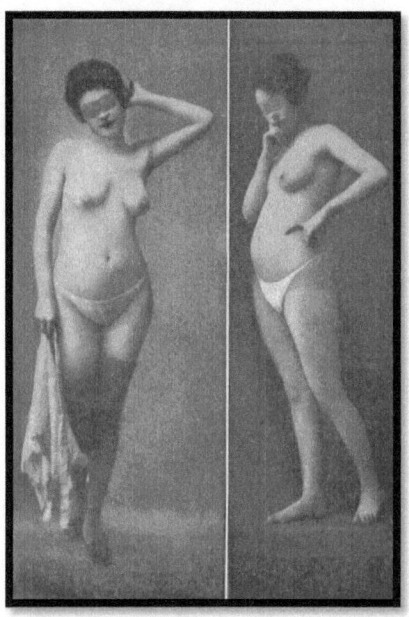

COMMON ALTERATION OF SHAPES

CONSEQUENCE OF INSUFFICIENT MUSCULAR DEVELOPMENT

Soft stomach and swollen, without muscular definition. Frail limbs, angular shoulders. Breasts in early third stage of sagging.

These women are considered well-built once corseted and dressed, with an absence of fat giving them a certain leanness.

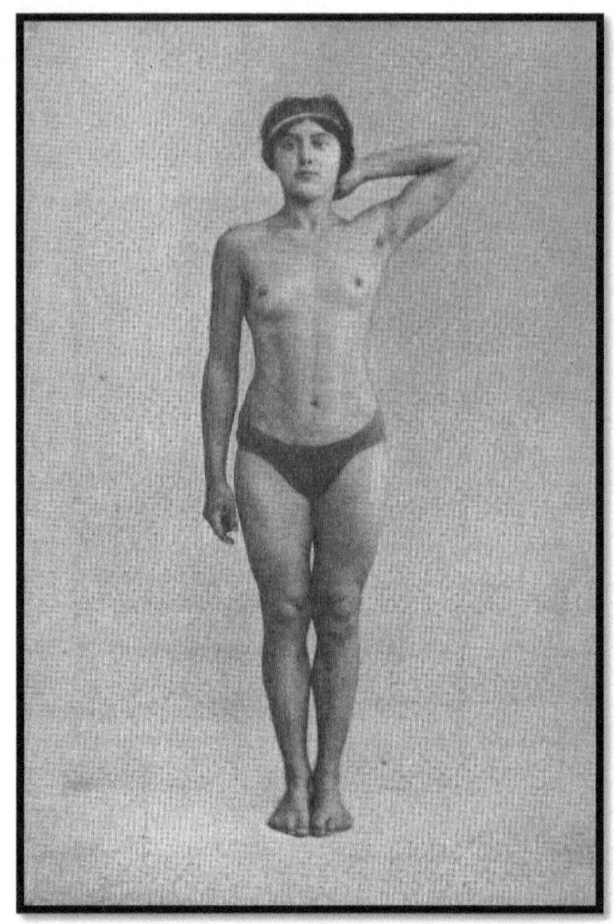

NORMALLY DEVELOPED INDIVIDUAL

Serving as comparison to the photo on the left.

Simple pose, unflattering for a woman, as it instantly shows defects of trunk and limbs.

Note: impeccable lower limbs line, big toes touching, remarkable definition of the abdominals, upper body development, solid arms, nice build.

# 30. IMPORTANCE OF THE DEVELOPMENT OF THE ABDOMINAL MUSCLES FOR HEALTH, BEAUTY AND STRENGTH.

The importance of abdominal muscles is capital, from an esthetics standpoint, as well as from strength and health standpoints.

When their development is insufficient, the abdominal belt is soft and mushy. There is a risk of herniation as a result of any effort, even of low intensity, after a fall, a simple misstep, a coughing spell, etc.

The internal organs (stomach, liver, intestines) improperly supported collapse under their own weight and make the belly protrude. The more this protrusion is pronounced, the more out of place the internal organs are in relation to their normal position. The resulting swelling render any effort hazardous.

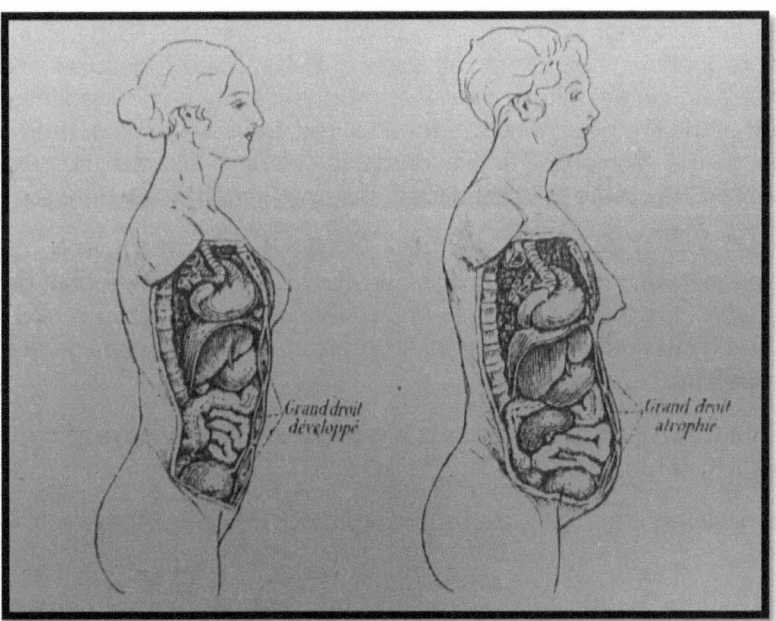

Figure 38. Dire consequences of the insufficiency of the abdominal musculature: poor placement of the internal organs. Left: normally developed abdominal muscles. The liver, stomach, kidneys are maintained in their normal position thanks to the firmness of the abdominal wall. Right: sagging belly. The internal organs are no longer in their normal position and their incorrect placement is the cause of many aches and pains.

Severe constipation, without success from medical prescriptions or pharmaceutical drugs, sometimes has no other cause than weakness in the abdominal musculature, or a simple lack of muscular training in that area, which helps promote waste elimination.

Breathing movements are always incomplete if the straight abdominals, exhaling muscles by excellence, are weak.

A woman's most important natural act, childbirth, is all the more facilitated that the abdominal muscles are powerfully developed.

As we just mentioned, not only do these muscles provide a shield for the anterior section of the body from ribs to iliac crest, but, additionally, any effort, be it pulling, pushing, lifting, etc., activates them more or less. Natural actions themselves: forced exhale, coughing, sneezing, shouting, defecation and finally childbirth, cannot occur without their engagement.

The future mother who keeps her abdominals "in shape" can continue well into her pregnancy, without risk, all sorts of natural and functional exercises, just like females in animal species. Her pregnant belly is reduced in volume, as a result of the firmness of her abdominal belt. Delivery is produced with extreme ease, in the fashion of active primitive women, without the necessity of a midwife. She is able to immediately resume her activities. Her stomach suffers no misshaping.

Abdominal weakness, by contrast, produces excessive pregnant belly volume. Any work or training becomes impossible early on, because of the nuisance caused by the belly's distension. A simple walk often causes great fatigue. Any intense effort is dangerous.

Childbirth, in that case, is painful; it necessitates many days of bed rest for the organs to settle back in.

After delivery, the belly remains distended, like an empty sack, with stretch marks.

Such is the physical inferiority of the civilized woman, inactive with no abdominal muscles, in relation to her primitive counterpart. When she delivers a child, she is treated as if she were ill. The natural act becomes delicate and dangerous instead of being "easy" and safe.

In Antique statues, the power of the abdominal muscles is striking in men as in women. The abdomen is a true muscular fortress. Sculptors understood the capital importance of these muscles, and their work proves they were considered like the primary attributes of health, beauty and strength. [PIX]

We can say that in civilized societies, the abdominal muscles of men, like women, have become weaker and weaker as the practice of natural and functional exercises, which would develop them, dropped: throwing, climbing, etc. The wearing of corsets, among women, has been a new cause of abdominal weakness.

Several generations will be needed, through training, before we can see the return of remarkable and powerful musculatures seen on Antique statues, especially when it comes to oblique muscles. Only a few athletes have such perfect development.

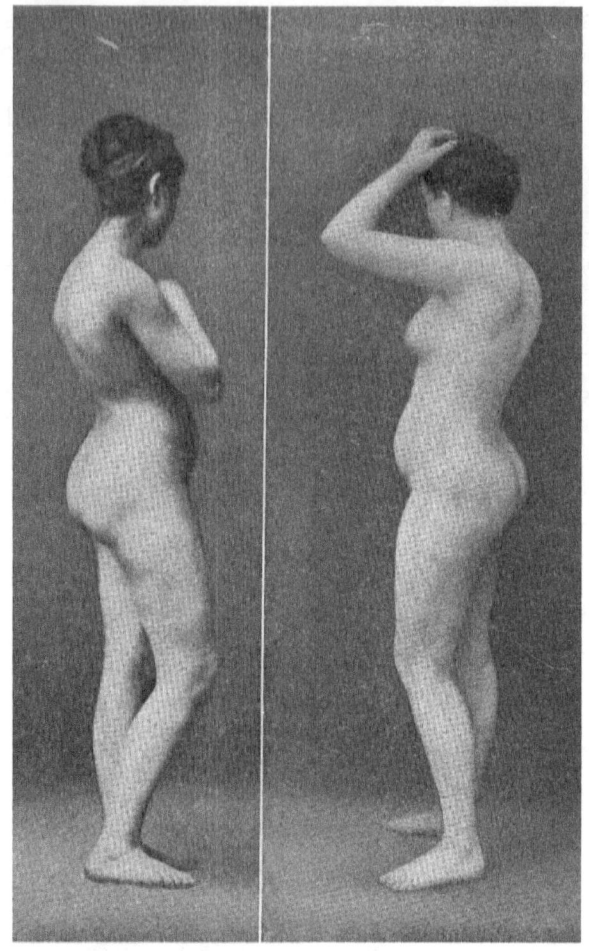

ALTERATION OF THE ABDOMINAL LINE RESULTING FROM INSUFFICIENT MUSCULAR
DEVELOPMENT

Two artist's models seemingly well-built as they are "filled" with a layer of fat
replacing absent muscles. Swollen bellies, slight saddling and slouched back on the
left subject. Compare her to the Venus of Milo, holding a similar pose.

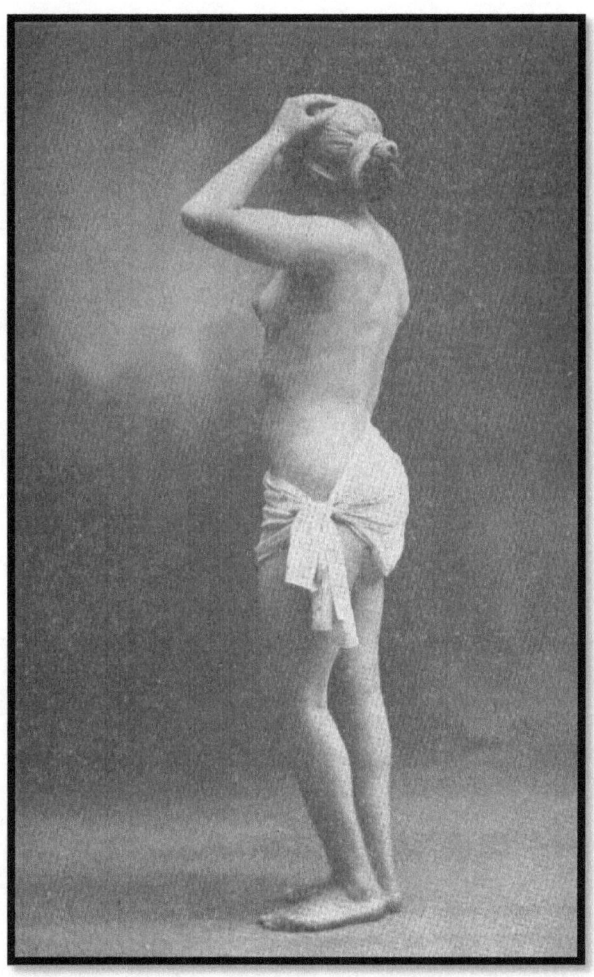

NORMAL ABDOMINAL LINE IN A FULLY DEVELOPED INDIVIDUAL

(Author's student)

Pose allowing the comparative study of body shape with the individuals on the left panel.

## 31. COMMON ABDOMINAL DEFORMITIES IN NON-DEVELOPED WOMEN.

The changes in the shape of the abdomen come, on one hand, from insufficient muscular development, and on the other hand, from the accumulation of fat tissue, or both combined.

In the case of insufficient muscular development without excess fat deposit, the stomach displays on of the following three aspects:

- ◉ *Swollen* all over, with a regular, yet convex line when viewed from the side.

- ◉ *Bloated* or swollen only in the lower portion, between the belly button and the pubis, with a profile line that's nearly circular between these two points.

- ◉ *Hanging* or *sagging*, with a pronounced profile line or slightly angular of the lower section.

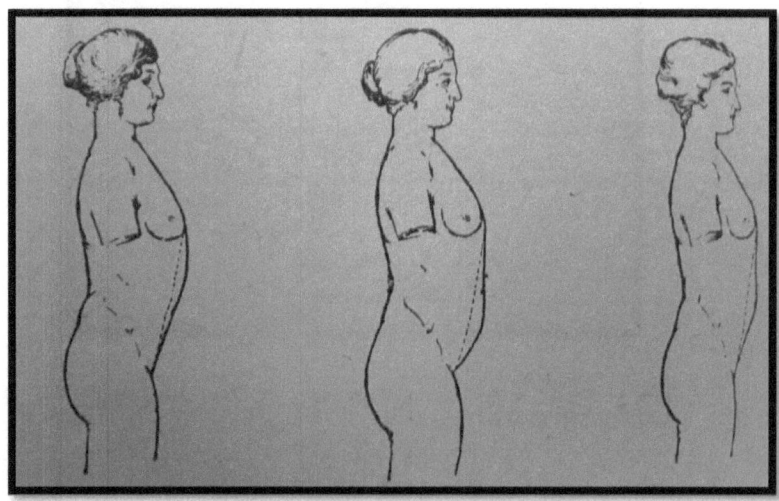

Figure 39. Abdominal deformities resulting from insufficient muscular development. Left: overall swollen stomach. Center: bottom swelling or rounding. Right: Sagging belly. The swollen or bloated bellies gradually turn into sagging bellies. The dotted line shows the normal abdominal line.

In the case of excess fat deposit, the stomach displays other aspects:

◉ When the fat is evenly spread out, the stomach is swollen, like in the first case described above, with the difference that it is hard to the touch, instead of being soft and mushy.

◉ When the fat is simply deposited between the sternum and the navel, it is swollen in the upper area. Its profile view presents a strong convex line in that spot. It's the *fatty upper belt line.*

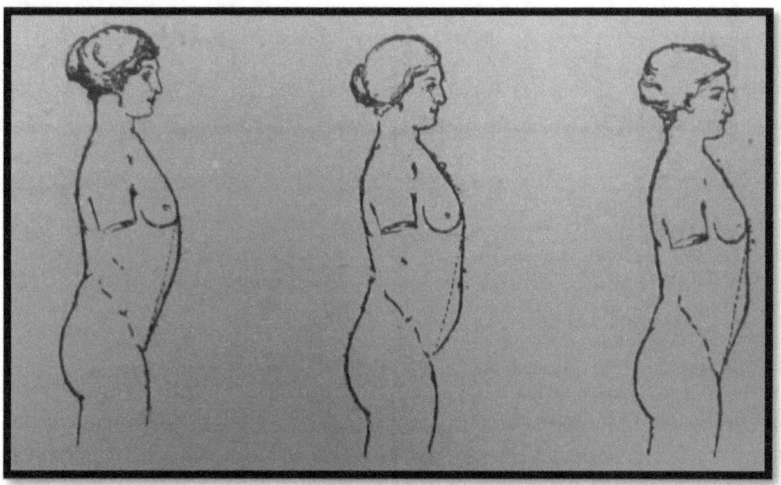

Figure 40. Deformity of the abdomen as a result of fat accumulation. Left: upper fatty belt. Center: lower fatty belt. Right: umbilical fatty belt, or umbilical bump/roll (frequent). The dotted line shows the normal line of the abdomen.

◉ When the fact, on the contrary, is between the navel and the pubis, it is swollen in its lower area. The profile view then presents a strong convex shape in the lower belly. It's the *fatty lower belt line.*

◉ When the fat is at or around belly button level, it is swollen at the waist. Its profile view is convex at the navel. This is the *fatty median belt line* or *umbilical,* or simply the *umbilical bump.*

◉ When the fat is accumulating both above and below the navel, it displays two swollen areas, and its profile view has two curves. This is called the *double fatty belt line.*

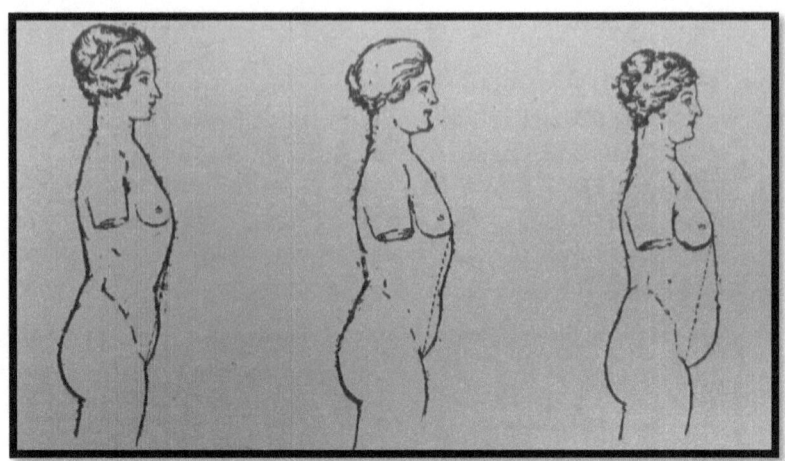

Figure 41. Other deformities of the abdomen. Left: hollowed, caved-in stomach, resulting from too much squeezing of the waist, particularly during childhood or adolescence. Center: double fatty belt, also a consequence of waist squeezing. Right: obesity. The dotted line shows the normal abdominal line.

When the accumulation of fat is combined with insufficient muscular development, the abdomen displays the most bizarre shape deviations. Thus, a sagging, fat-overloaded stomach in the lower belly, hangs completely over the pubis.

In all cases of insufficient muscular development or fat accumulation, however small it may be, muscular definition is always absent and the shape of the muscles invisible. The stomach is smooth/soft, even during contraction. [PIC]

When the trunk is flexed forward or laterally, abnormal rolls appear on a fat stomach, mainly on the sides, above the hips.

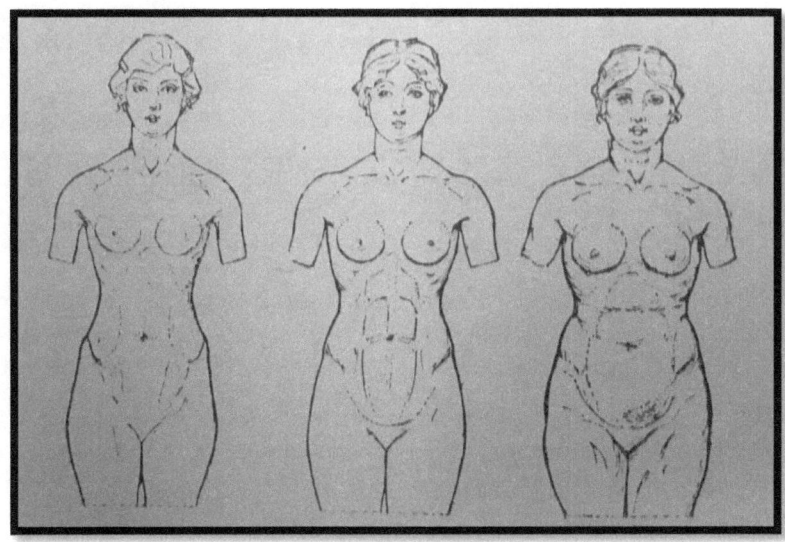

Figure 42. Lateral abdominal deformity of the waist and disappearance of the normal shape of the abdomen by either lack of muscular development or excess fat deposit. Center: normal shape of the waist, normal development of the rectus abdominis and the obliques. Left: deformity resulting from insufficient muscular development. The hip bones are jutting out, muscular definition/shape is absent, and the stomach is flat. Right: deformity due to excess fat deposits. The belly is swollen, covered in fat and smooth.

In addition, skin folds and stretch marks hide the abdomen from one hip to the other.

On many modern sculptures, we can see some of these deficiencies, especially a smooth, swollen belly with a fatty bump at the navel or rolls on the sides ("love handles").

# CHAPTER VI : THE BREASTS AND THEIR DEFORMITIES

## 32. DISTINCTION TO ESTABLISH BETWEEN THE CHEST AND THE BREASTS. BEAUTY OF THE CHEST'S SHAPE.

In common speak, women often used the same word to describe two different body parts: the chest and the breasts. The chest simply serves as a base of support for the breasts; its beauty is completely distinct from the latter.

Well-conformed breasts can exist on an underdeveloped chest, muscularly or with poor bone structure (flat chest or rounded chest), and inversely, deformed breasts can often be positioned on a nice chest. The chest extends from the clavicles to the lower part of the thorax. Its best conformation, from a point of view of bone structure, has been indicated in Chapter III.

The chest is filled with the muscle of the *pectorals* and the *serratus*; the beauty of its shape depends mostly on the development of the pectoralis major.

The pectorals link the humerus (funny bone) to the clavicle, the ribs and the sternum; in other words, they cover the entire upper portion of the thorax. Their mass makes up the anterior edge of the armpit.

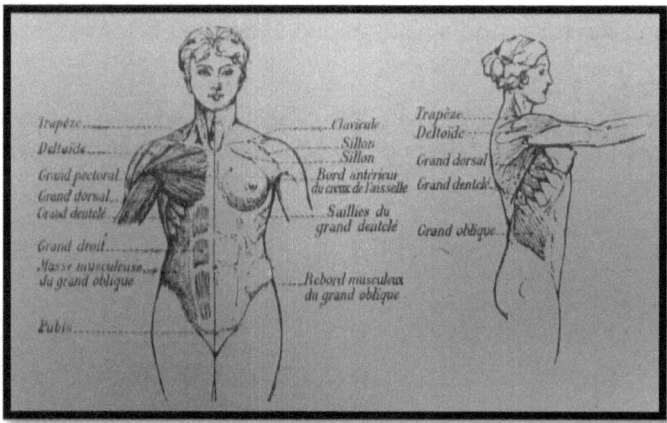

Figure 43. Anatomical and plastic study of the chest and abdomen. On the left, the right side of the body is showed "skinned", the left side shows the various lines of the muscular shape an visible contours on a naked body with perfect development.

They activate during traction created by the arms, forward, backwards, high and low; in hanging by the hands, climbing or in any effort of closing or bringing the arms closer to one another.

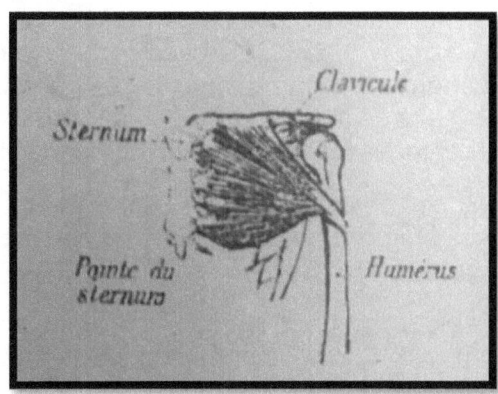

Figure 44. The Pectoralis Major. The beauty in the shape of the chest depends greatly on the development of the pectoral muscle. This muscle, which constitutes the anterior edge of the armpit, serves as an attachment base for the breast.

In perfect development, when the arms are very close together, when the pectorals are maximally contracted, the internal edges of their curves are defined as a groove with sinuous edges. Also, two slightly curved lines (inter-muscular grooves) appear under the clavicles and form a large upside down V across the chest; two other lines, also curved (pectoral-deltoid grooves) are drawn at the meeting of the pectorals and deltoid muscles [PIC]. Finally, a little gap, like a dimple, appears on the edge of the armpit, near the breast.

In the case of insufficient pectoral development, the anterior edge of the armpit is without thickness. When contracted, it forms no sharp edge and shows no hardness. An ugly depression forms near the shoulder, just above the armpit.

This dent is common among all women having never done upper body training. The accumulation of fat often fills that, but it reappears at the first signs of weight loss.

Atrophy of the pectoral muscles makes the upper thorax appear void of muscle. The ribs can be seen through the skin, above the breasts; clavicles are strongly jutting, unless fat filled this area.

The serratus, of which only a portion is visible, fills the lower lateral part of the thorax. It connects the shoulder blade to the ribs, and, like the trapezius, maintains that bone flat on the thorax. [PIC]

It activates in nearly all pulling movements, or pushing, of the upper limbs and more specifically in raising the arms overhead, hanging by the hands and various climbing efforts. Its shape is more visible when the arms are elevated. It can be then seen as a series of short superimposed rolls, five in number, the first three quite apparent and over the edge of the thorax.

In perfectly developed cases, these muscular rolls are extremely hard when contracted. Those not knowledgeable in the human shape think they are ribs jutting out, pitying the person for being so seemingly skinny.

The serratus is visible only among women who worked climbing exercises and have no fat accumulation. Its development goes hand in hand with that of the arms, back, chest and abdominal muscles. This muscle is a criterion: its shape alone can help judge the degree of general muscular trunk development.

[PIX]

## 33. THE BREASTS. NORMAL AND DEFECTIVE SHAPES.

The breasts are not made up of muscles, but glands, mammary glands, which have their insertion point directly on the pectoral muscles. Their robustness and firmness is as a result dependent in most part on the power of these muscles, which serve both as a support base, as well as anchor point.

To properly take this dependence in consideration, one only needs to raise the arms overhead or strongly retract the shoulders back. The pectorals, by stretching, immediately straighten the breasts up considerably.

A normally conformed breast presents all the following characteristics: [PICS]

⊙ Relatively small volume and low on weight;

⊙ Possesses a certain firmness to the touch and adheres well to the skin;

⊙ Its general shape is that of a spherical cap.

Seen from the front, its outer contour is circular. The nipple, or breast tip, is at equal distance from all the points from the base contour.

The thickness of the breast or its maximal prominence measure from the side (nipple height projected above the sub-mammary region) and is equal to half the width or diameter of the base. As a practical indicator, the breast's owner should be able to entirely cover it with their hand, fingers spread maximally, with the fingertips touching the outer edge.

The breast detaches from the chest without a brusque transition and appears, in its upper half, one with that muscle.

The line that draws its contour is barely visible in the upper and lateral internal parts; it is only pronounced in the lower external part, in other words the lowest edge of the pectoral muscles (or a quarter of the entire contour, approximately).

No skin fold should show on the lower contour.

From a profile view, the trunk upright and chest open, the contour line is convex and somewhat circular, with the exception of the nipple.

The line that joins the nipples goes above the arch of the sternum. This arch or upper part of the epigastric dip is well above the tip of the sternum, exactly at the beginning of the last rib cartilage.

Between the breasts is a groove ample enough that the internal sinuous edges of the pectorals are visible when contracted, and not covered by the breasts. [PIC]

The nipples point horizontally, slightly out or to the side, when the trunk is vertical.

Finally, during walking, running jumping and generally during any displacement exercises, the breasts, unsupported by any bra or corset, cause no discomfort, in other words, their swaying isn't bothersome, if normal in volume and weight, are well-anchored and closely adhere to the skin.

Poorly conformed breasts, or deformed, display the following aspects:

◉ *Atrophy*, when their development is insufficient in relation to the age and general body proportions;

◉ *Hypertrophy*, when on the contrary their development in volume is exaggerated, also in relation to the body proportions or age. Hypertrophy can also be excessive.

◉ *Skinny*, flat or as saucers, when their thickness or prominence is inferior to normal standards previously mentioned.

◉ *Large* or spread out, when the base diameter is too wide.

◉ *Narrow*, when the base diameter is too small.

◉ *Bouncy* or apple-shaped, when their convex surface is exaggerated in the upper portion.

◉ *Elongated* or pear-shaped, when their general shape is like a cone instead of being spherical.

◉ *Spread apart*, when there are positioned on the sides of the chest, so that the nipples point outward or the gap between them is exaggerated.

◉ *Close together* or tangent, when positioned on the middle of the chest, with nipples pointing straight forward or inward, and when their internal edges touch or the gap separating them is too narrow.

◉ *Seated low*, when the line joining the nipples is level with, or lower than sternum height.

◉ *In the air*, when the nipples point above horizontal.

◉ *Fat*, swollen or ballooned up, filled only with fat deposits.

◉ *Mushy*, when they present no firmness.

◉ *Poorly anchored or swaying*, when they sway at every movement.

◉ *Asymmetrical*, when they are not of the same shape or placed differently.

- *Pointy,* when the areolas, or base of the areolas, detach from the breast proper and present a conic shape.

- *Sagging* or *hanging,* when the nipples are no longer equidistant from the outer edges of the breasts' base.

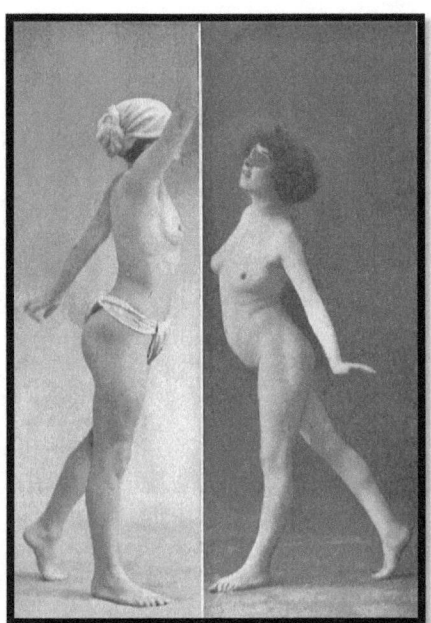 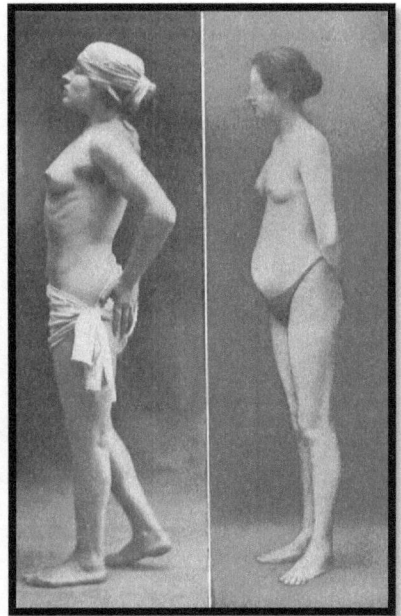

**NORMAL ABDOMINAL SHAPE AND MOST COMMON FORM DEVIATIONS**

*Far Left:* Normal abdominal shape of the abdomen in a fully developed individual (author's student).

*Second from left:* swollen belly, light saddling, flat thorax, fat rolls on the flanks, skinny arms, breasts in second stage of sagging.

*Second from right:* normal abdominal line in a fully developed individual (author's student).

*Far right:* strongly swollen belly, flat thorax, angular shoulders, and frail limbs.

## 34. THE THREE STAGES OF BREAST SAGGING.

Sagging breasts can be seen in various aspects depending on the degree of sagging achieved. Their deformity is progressive, is made up of three main phases or stages until complete drop.

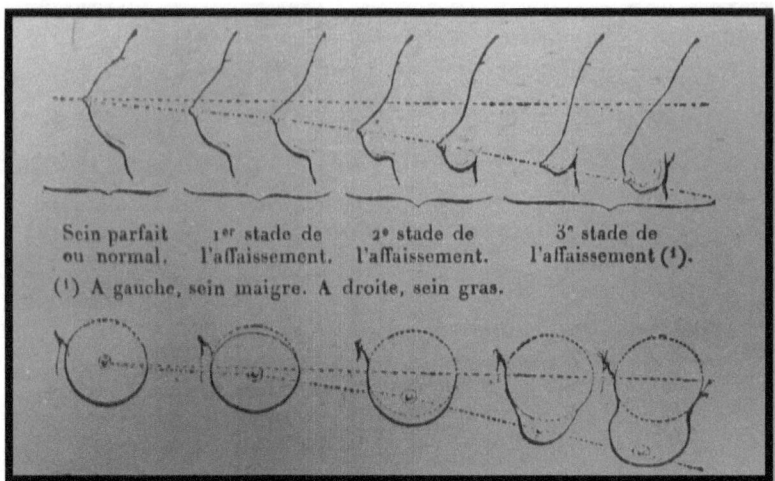

Figure 45. The three stages of breast sagging. On the bottom drawings, the circular dotted line indicates the normal contour of the breast. Top: breast line from side view. Bottom: External contour of the breast, frontal view. At the first stage, the upper breast line from side view is straight or slightly concave. The nipple is only slightly off-center. At the second stage, the upper breast line from a side view is concave. Frontally, the lower contour of the breast is hidden by the breast itself. Third stage: the nipple is near the bottom of the breast. The breast is flattened if skinny or swollen if overweight.

For the following description, the body is assumed to be in a proper upright stance, the entire back against a wall, from heels to back of head.

At the first stage of sagging, the nipple is barely displaced from its normal position, but the breasts' upper portion flattens and its contour seen from the side becomes nearly a straight line. The lower part slightly increases in volume and convexity; finally, the lower contour becomes more pronounced.

At the second stage, the nipple is clearly off-center, meaning below its normal position. The upper half of the breast continues to flatten while the lower half increases in volume and convexity. Its profile line is straight, sometimes even concave in its upper half, and of a very pronounced convexity in its lower half.

The most important characteristic of this second stage is the following: from the front, the lower contour is no longer visible; it is covered by the breast itself. Additionally, a skinfold forms at the contour's spot.

At the third stage, the drop is complete. *The nipple is placed in the lower portion of the breast.* All of the mammary's flesh seems to have dropped into the lower portion of the breast like into the bottom of a pocket. Depending on whether the breast is fat or skinny, its shape is that of a full or nearly empty pocket.

When the trunk is leaned forward, instead of upright, the breast, even normal, hangs, as a result of this movement and under its own weight, this appearing like the first stage of the sagging. In other words, the upper portion of the breast sags slightly and its profile contour is a straight line.

It is very important to note that this is not a deformity, rather a change of state that only results from a shifting in position of the body. So is the *Venus of Milo*, whose upper body is leaning forward and whose breasts depict this particularity.

Let's add, to complete this explanation, that breasts that truly are in the first stage of sagging when the body is in a correct upright stance, immediately shift into the second stage when the trunk is leaned forward.

The shape of the breast in the first stage can be considered normal in a fully developed woman, especially if she breastfed. This shape is still beautiful and not frequent. It's the shapes of the second and third stages that we encounter most often.

The shape of the breasts is considered wrongly by many as a criterion of beauty in a woman. "The breasts, that the whole woman", we have heard in stupid refrains. In reality, the shape of the breasts only makes up one element of general beauty, and its importance is only secondary when compared to essential body parts: the abdomen, the chest, the limbs, etc.

It is, if we may, one of the first attributes of beauty among young women, but not in the adult woman, as of all her attributes, it's the least durable.

This process, a little too simplistic, which consists of judging the beauty of a woman according to the shape of her breasts comes without a doubt from the following fact: on an under-developed trunk, skinny or fat, the breasts first catch the eye, because, as a rule, these organs present defects of which the most common ones are exaggerated volume and sagging. They thus appear to have a capital importance, because their misshaping alone breaks the general harmony of the body.

On a well-developed trunk, on the contrary, with well-defined muscles, normal breasts barely get any attention.

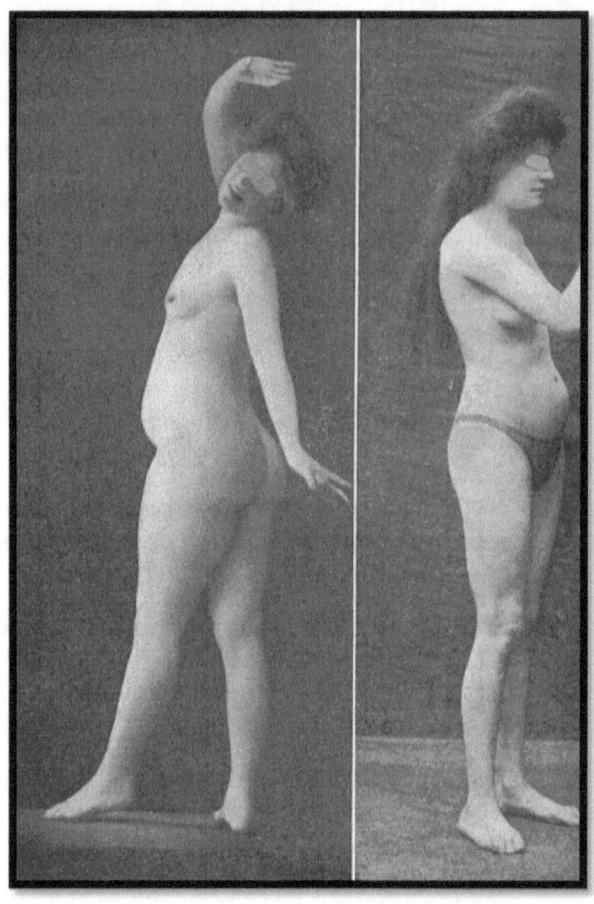

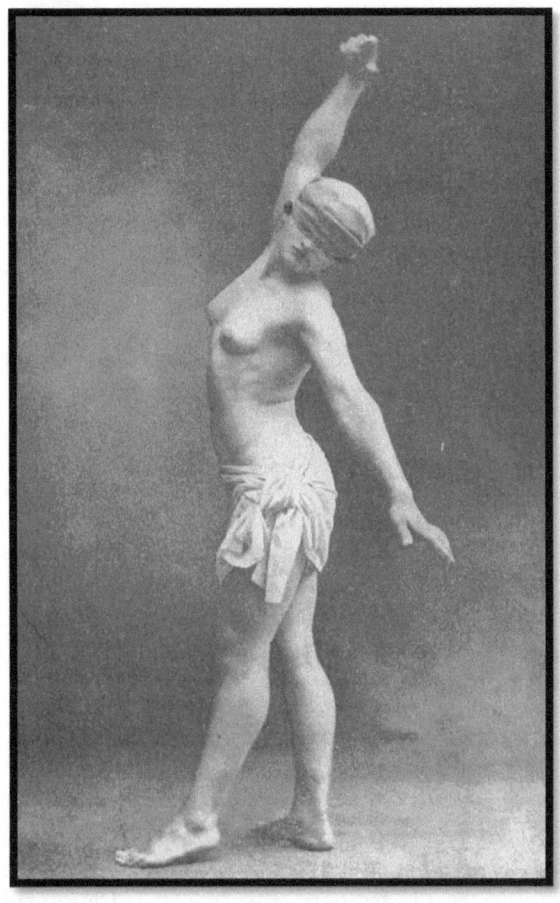

NORMAL SHAPE AND ITS ALTERATION FROM INSUFFICIENT MUSCULAR DEVELOPMENT

Comparative study of the shape of an athlete (author's student) and two non-developed individuals, with frail limbs, flat thorax, sagging breasts and swollen belly.

They are well molded onto the chest and solidly anchored to the pectorals that they look as if being entirely part of these muscles. In the preceding case, they seem added to the chest, which seemed inconvenienced to carry them.

The same observation could be applied to the basin and buttocks, which always appear too big when the trunk is muscularly atrophied.

## 35. CAUSES FOR THE SAGGING OF BREASTS.

The breasts lose their firmness, shape and drop under the influence of various causes, of which the main ones are:

1) At first, lack of physical exercise, which results in the flesh becoming soft and without tone. The breasts suffer the repercussions of this general softening.

2) Poor general health or simply fragile health, frailty, anemia… In other words, any state of weakening of the body.

3) Poor general posture.

   With a good posture, the internal wall of the chest is inclined, as we discussed previously, at an angle of about 45°. In this case, the breast rests on an oblique base: part of its weight is supported by the base. If, at the same time, the shoulder is back, it is then lifted and supported by the pectoral muscle.

   With improper posture or a person lets themselves go, on the contrary, the chest flattens and its internal wall is vertical, or almost vertical. The breast rests on a very inclined base or drops. Its weight, if higher than normal, pulls the ligaments that anchor it and presses the skin more strongly than when the chest is properly positioned. If at the same time the shoulder rolls forward, the breast is lowered by a relaxing of the pectoral muscle, which increases the pull under its own weight.

   The importance of a good posture is thus capital in the conservation of the shape of the breast, when the latter is of a considerable weight.

4) Insufficiently developed pectoral muscles.

5) Lack of tonicity or elasticity in the skin.

A loose or non-elastic skin extends easily under pressure or pulling, but does not tighten or only returns to its original state imperfectly. When the skin presents this condition, the breasts progressively start to droop by simply stretching the skin that covers them with their own weight.

This is a common occurrence and presents no remedy.

6) The continuous wear of a brassiere or of a high corset.

A general rule of physiology teaches us that any device that replaces the action of any organ, such as a muscle or a ligament, forces it into inaction and weakens it over time.

When the ligaments that attach the breasts are routinely replaced by a bra or corset, they progressively atrophy.

After a while, they lose all resistance. As soon as the support device is removed, the breasts drop, especially when heavy, or the skin lost its elasticity and the support device was used for a long time.

The bra should only be an orthopedic device designed to support hypertrophied, deformed or sagging breasts. The majority of women instead treat it as an indispensable accessory to wear continuously, as early as adolescence. Some would not part with it under any circumstances, even when choosing to exercise. They believe that physical exercise, especially running or jumping, by shaking their breasts, unavoidably cause breast sagging when in reality, it only strengthens and tones them up. Such is the current common knowledge.

Could we believe, for instance, that there are models for painters and sculptors who, imbued with this preconceived notion, are advised by artists as ignorant as themselves, to be condemned to lie down and stretch themselves as much as possible and live in a way as to avoid any movement, even a car ride, to preserve the shape of their breasts intact?! Isn't that the ultimate misbelief of the fragile nature of the doll-woman?

7) An exaggerated development from birth. This defect, when not caused by excess fat tissue, is impossible to make go away.

8) Repeated breast-feeding and also age. These natural causes can be stalled as long as full physical development and activity are maintained.

9) Finally, because of excess fat deposit, which is the most common cause of drooping.

We have already indicated in previous chapters the frequency of the overload of fat tissue in women, as a result of lack of physical exercise generally associated to either irrational or exaggerated food intake.

Observation shows that the breasts are, with the abdomen, the body parts where fat tends to unfortunately accumulate.

Many adolescent and young adults carry, precociously, breasts that are full, enveloped in excess fat rapidly and completely. Unfortunately, this is brief. Under the fat, with growing up, the breasts fill up even more until reaching a point where they exceed their natural development.

As we mentioned it already, a well-formed breast is not only small, but also light in weight. Or, with an increase in volume due to excess fat comes an increase in weight. Under the resulting excess pressure coming on one hand from the increase in volume, and on the other hand an increase in weight, the skin covering the breasts distends slowly, regardless of its degree of tonicity. The breasts drop and flatten on their upper part and sags, taking the shape of a pocket.

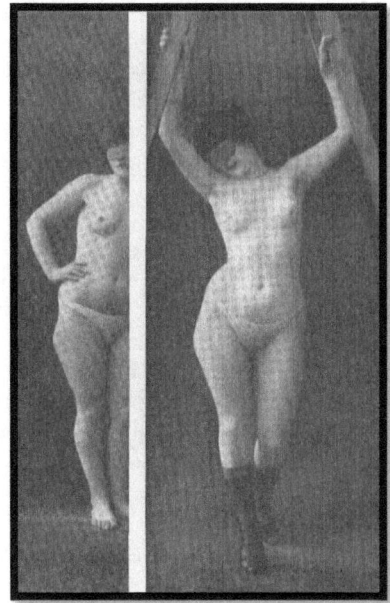 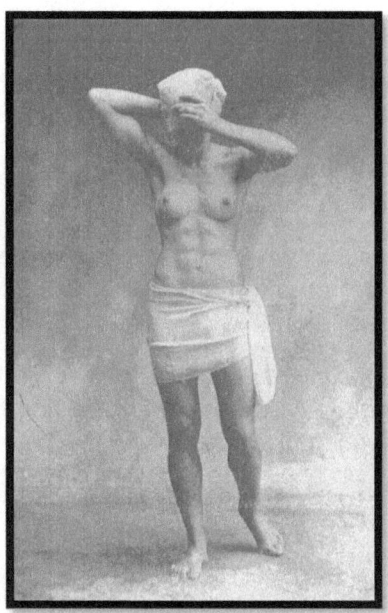

NATURAL WAISTLINE AND CORSET DEFORMATION

CORSET DEFORMED WAIST

Right of left panel: angular waistline, flat hips.

Left: rolls on thighs coming from excess fat deposit redistributed by the squeezing from a corset. Among heavier individuals, the squeezing redistributes the fat to the basin, which expands the hips.

Right Panel: Normal waist shape in a fully developed individual (author's student) in a pose serving to compare her with the subjects on the left panel.

Notice the perfect definition of the abdominal and oblique muscles, the definition in the pectorals between the breasts.

Young individuals with excess fat can have breasts with an attractive appearance so long as the skin remains tight. But this doesn't last and sagging occurs at the latest between the ages of 23 and 25. With a stronger fat deposit, breasts can begin to sag as early as age 14 or 15, even earlier, if the skin gives in.

At any age, as a result of excess fat inflating the breasts and seemingly giving them a firm look, when weight loss takes place, even a return to a normal state, a sagging of the breasts is inevitable. The fat being gone, the distended skin only returns to its shape in part, or not at all if its elasticity is weak.

In summary, excess weight and volume coming from a fat overload, bring about the dropping of the breasts.

Based on what was said about the filling of the breasts resulting from excess fat deposit, we can guess the tricks of snake-oil salesmen pretending to have the solution to firm breasts.

The products they offer have no other purpose than to fatten up their clients or simply give them appetite. Since fat as a tendency to choose the breasts as one of its first hosts, the predicted result is thus achieved. The breasts indeed firm up or size up because they fill with fat. At the first sign of weight loss, the sagging will only be more pronounced.

Many women believe in the effectiveness or cold water ablutions to maintain or regain tone in their breasts. Upon contact with water, especially cold water, the skin firms up and tightens up. This is true for any part of the body. But this skin tonicity only lasts a few moments, the water having only a negligible action on the firming of the mammary glands.

# CHAPTER VII : NATURAL WAIST AND ITS DEFORMING BY CORSETS

## 36. JUDGMENT REGARDING A THIN WAIST AND THE FASHION OF THE CORSET.

The waistline's beauty can only result from the integral development and the maintenance and conditioning of the muscles of the abdominal region.

A waistline is beautiful when it is natural and not when it is atrophied, with excess fat deposits or misshaped by voluntary compression.

It is, as we saw in Chapter II, the ignorance of the normal human shape and the abandonment of physical exercise, from which the preconceived notion of a thin waist was born and brought about the trend of squeezing into a corset.

It seems almost superfluous, after all we have said regarding beauty or health, to warn against the setbacks of corsets and the damages such a device can create, especially one whose only function is to modify natural shapes and encroach on the free motion of internal organs. But, how could we not insist?

No argument, indeed, no suffering even, has been effective in having women reject such a ridiculous torture device, only to restrict its usage. Quite the contrary, those who object themselves to this forced squeezing grow in numbers daily in many countries. From cities, corsets have slowly penetrated the farthest countryside.

Countrywomen begin by wearing corsets on market days or for parties. Nearly all housekeepers coming from the country and placed for work in cities would feel ashamed if their waistline weren't bound tightly. In city schools, the majority of young girls, even from poor families, are already adorning a corset starting at the age of ten!

This weird and hazardous fashion is spreading around the globe like an epidemic. It is a true plague, which doesn't spare exotic countries. What traveler hasn't met one day a rich indigenous corseted woman, in areas where clothing is only of secondary importance, considering the warm local weather!

Corset makers spread their merchandise everywhere. They usually have no trouble convincing the most incredulous ones of the need to imprison one's trunk with their devices. They need only say: "that's the trend, everyone wears them!"

These words make up the supreme argument that no one seeks to contest. The woman then sacrifices everything, without hesitation, even her health, to satisfy this incredibly artificial beauty requirement.

Anyone with common sense agrees to condemn corsets. What we are about to discuss about the nefarious influence on health, beauty and strength of this compression device is not new. The dangers of squeezing the waistline have been brought to light for centuries, by many people; we are merely echoing them.

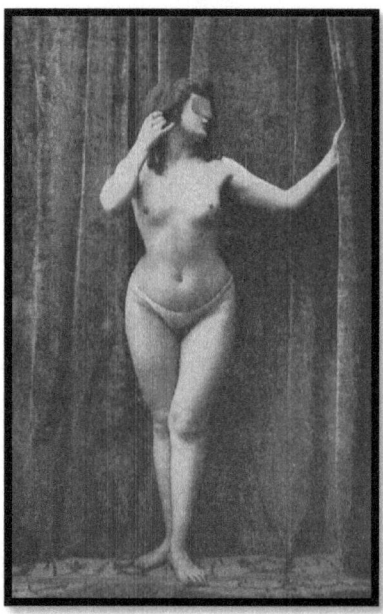 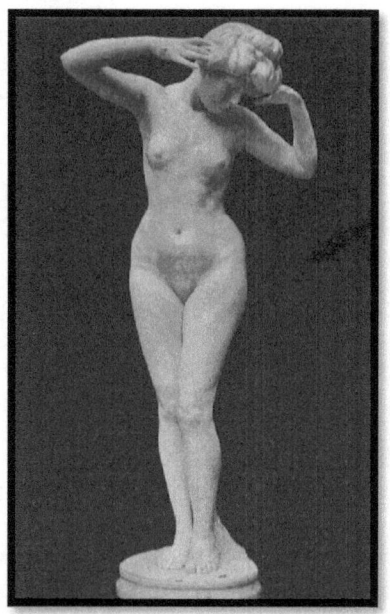

ALTERATION OF THE WAISTLINE BY CORSET

Comparative study of an individual whose waist was deformed by wearing corsets as well as modern art reproducing this deformity.

Left: individual presenting a deformation of the trunk by wearing a corset. The waistline has sharp angles.

Right: Nymph, artist: October (Luxembourg museum, Paris).

The deformation of the waist and shrinking of the lower part of the thorax are sharply accentuated. The muscular insufficiency of the trunk is apparent. Additionally, her big toes are deviated. These observations, relative to the shape of the depicted subject, in no way hinder the purely artistic value of this sculpture, full of charm and finesse.

## 37. DISADVANTAGES OF CORSETS ON HEALTH.

1) Wearing a corset from a young age stunts the proper growth of the thorax and restricts breathing capacity.

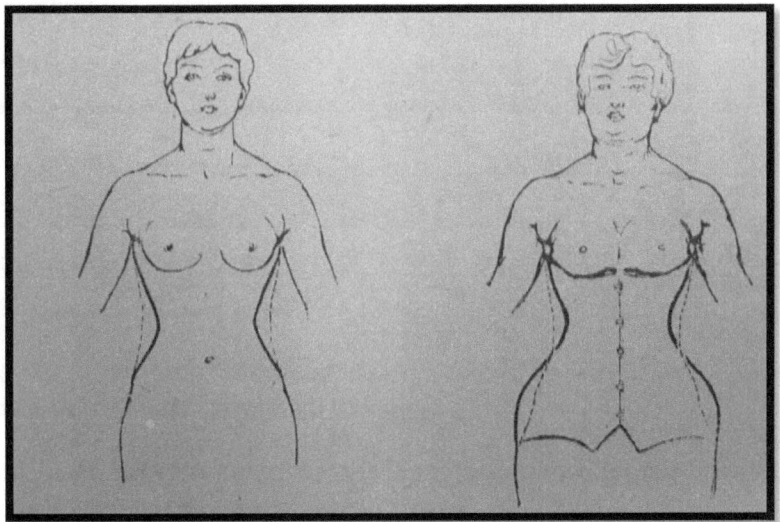

Figure 46. Waist deformation by corset wear. Left: most common deformation. Right: deformation in the case of excess body fat. The corset redistributes the fat deposits to the hips and thus increases the basin's amplitude. The dotted line indicates a natural waistline.

The young woman condemned to wear a corset becomes gradually crippled at the thoracic cage with atrophied lungs.

2) Corsets prevent the movement of expansion in the abdomen and the low ribs.

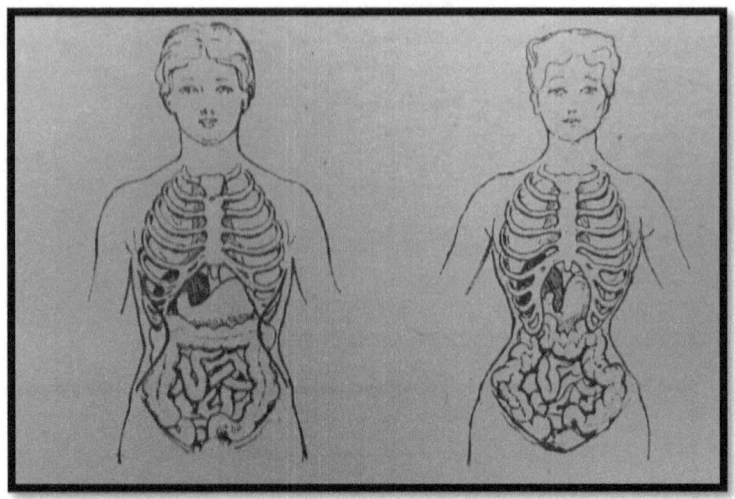

Figure 47. Side effects of corset wear on the internal organs. Left: natural waistline, normal position of internal organs and full thorax development. The darker line indicates the position of a corset and shows the organs it would forcefully reposition. Right: corset deformed waistline. Shrunken lower ribs, compressed internal organs pushed downward into the lower belly.

During normal breathing, without obstruction from clothing, the first beat of the inhale is noticeable by a forward push of the stomach, and the second beat by a lifting of the upper chest. The first movement, which allows a deep and complete penetration of air into the lower lungs, is rendered nearly impossible by the corset.

With a corset, the inhale occurring more or less only in the upper chest, the lungs are never filled completely.

However, the freer and ample the breathing, the more oxygenated blood is and is thus richer for nourishing tissue. On another hand, an incomplete breathing pattern causes breathlessness and makes any effort painful.

It's this way of breathing with the upper chest, a direct consequence of the encumbrance to the expansion of the lower ribs and the abdomen by the corset, which makes people (including doctors) believe or say that men breathe differently from women.

3)   The corset, by the simple pressure it causes on the trunk, produces a slowing down of circulation, which, consequently, prevents vital functions from being fully performed.

When an organ functions, it needs a greater amount of blood, circulation being more active in that area. If it doesn't receive an appropriate amount of blood, it functions poorly or partially.

4)   Corsets created a debilitating effect on the digestive organs.

To digest food well, the stomach cannot be compressed. After a meal, it needs to expand, not only because of what it ingested, but because it needs to freely execute the movements of *kneading* necessary to mix the digestive acids with the food.

The corset makes this important task difficult, or reduces it greatly. It also makes it impossible, or considerably reduces the *massage* of the stomach, liver and intestines by the diaphragmatic muscle, which, at every breathing movement, needs to go up and down with full amplitude.

Women being tightly squeezed, even with a belt, all suffer digestive troubles, without exception. Their stomach functions poorly, and their intestines become lazy.

5)   A corset, even when lightly laced, exercises a constant compression on the upper and lower abdomen. It is thus the cause of all kinds of sexual dysfunctions and organ displacements.

This setback was brought to an extreme with a trend twenty years ago, when the squeezing would take place at belt level, splitting the waist in two.

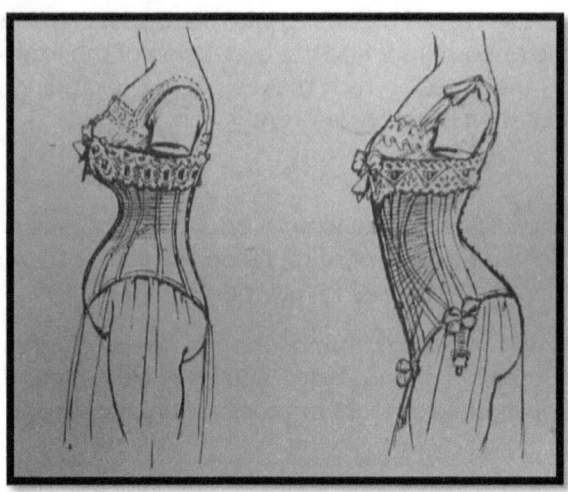

Figure 48. Abdominal and lumbar deformation by corset wear. Left: the corset as fashionable twenty years prior to original publication. The abdomen is cut in two, the bosom lifted and the belly strongly rounded. The lumbar curve remains relatively normal. Right: More recent corset fashion. Everything is "straight in front", sending everything to the back with a pronounced lumbar arch (lordosis).

With a corset called "straight forward", this still exists, even if to a lesser degree, despite what corset makers and corset defenders claim, among whom we can find doctors. The compression on the internal organs occurs *laterally* instead of *peripherally* as with older styles of corsets. However, one doesn't need to be an expert in mechanical science to understand that this new kind of compression leads to the same consequence on internal organs. In a seated position, the compression becomes the same as it was with the previous trend.

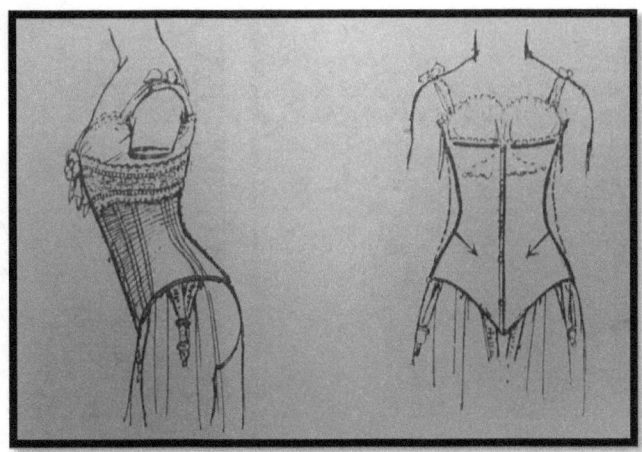

Figure 49. Latest corset trend. Side view: close to natural line, but from the front, we can instantly notice the pressure from tightening too much, just like in older corset fashions. On the right, the arrows indicate the direction of compression on the abdomen and the dotted line indicates a natural waistline.

In summary, to have a young woman wear a corset is to bring about irreparable organ disorders; it's a sentence to remain *fragile*.

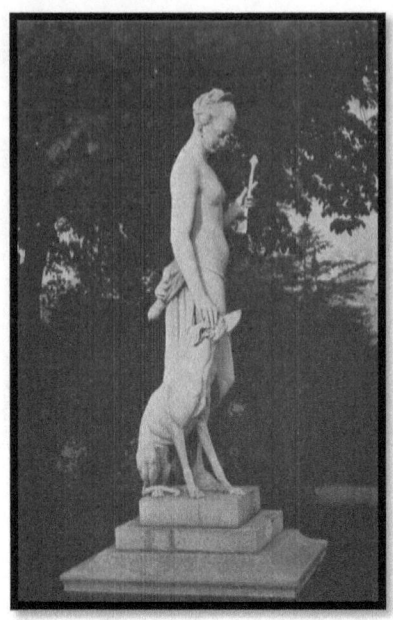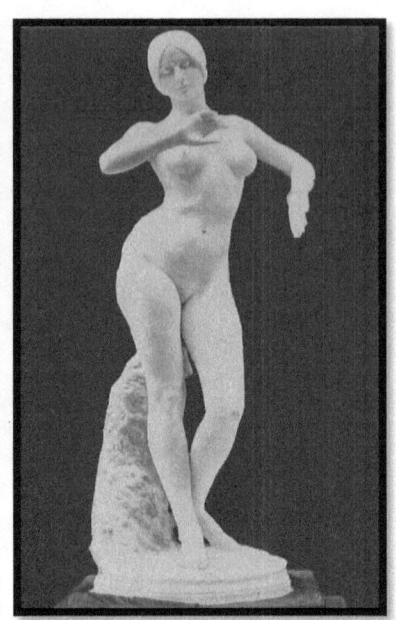

COMMON ABDOMINAL AND WAISTLINE ALTERATIONS REPRODUCED IN SCULPTURES.

Left: Diana, artist: Lévêque (Tuileries Gardens, Paris).

Example of sagging belly, insufficient muscular development, sloping shoulders.

Right: Dance, artist: Falguière.

Deformed waistline, soft stomach.

# 38. DISADVANTAGES OF CORSETS ON BEAUTY.

1) The corset produces deformities in the lower ribs and shrinks the lower part of the thorax.

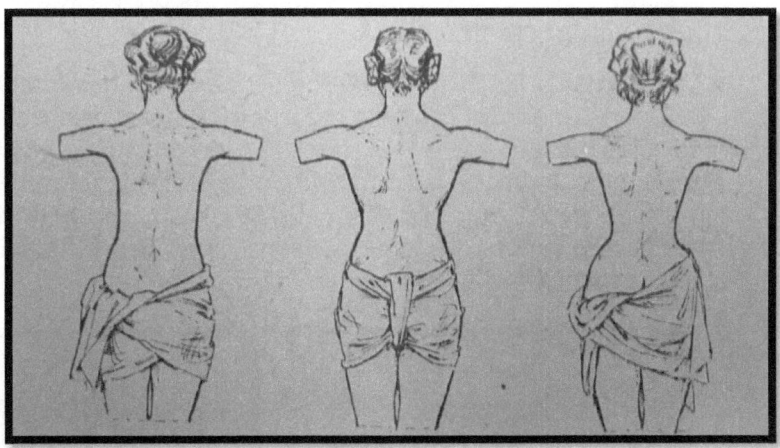

Figure 50. Waistline alterations from corset wear (back view). Center: normal V-shape from waist to armpits as a result of normal muscular development of the latissimus dorsi. Left: corset deformed back with cylindrical shape or nearly parallel sides resulting from insufficient muscular development of the "lats". This atrophied back becomes shaped like the drawing on the right when the waistline is deformed by the corset. Right: abnormal V-shape of an atrophied back too tightly squeezed by a corset.

The waistline, from armpit to hip, becomes angular at the narrowest part of the trunk.

2) The corset atrophies the abdominal muscles and the lumbar muscles.

We already indicated that when any device replaces the action of a muscle, that muscle, having nothing left to do, gradually weakens.

Corsets, well cinched at the waist and sitting on the hips, maintain by themselves the chest in vertical position; it replaces thus the balancing muscles of the torso, which are none other than the abdominals and the lumbar muscles.

Women who are constantly corseted have a swollen belly, hanging or protruding, as a result of the relaxing of the abdominal muscles. They usually have a smooth or flattened back, right above the basin, instead of having two sacral-lumbar muscular mounds extending from the spine. [PICS]

The woman who takes off her corset has the feeling that everything collapses. The older she gets, the more intense the sensation, because muscles weaken more and more. It even reaches a point where it is impossible to move around without a "stake", since the atrophied muscles no longer function naturally. Also, some women do not hesitate to emphasize their nonsensical stance by stating that "the corset is indispensable to women".

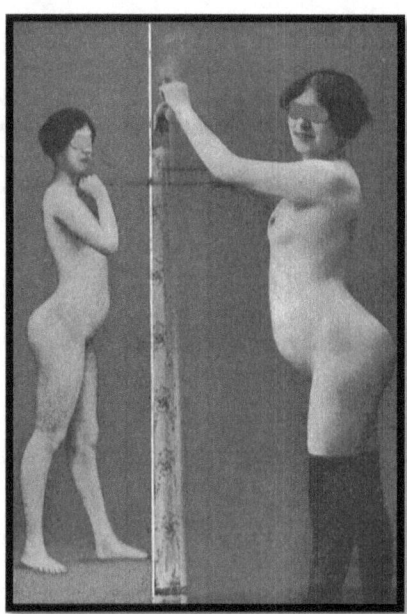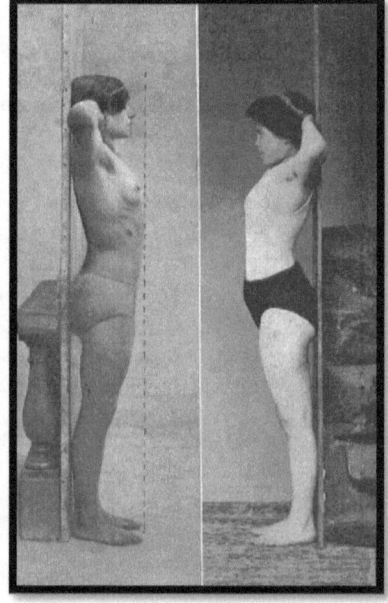

COMMON SHAPE ALTERATIONS

Saddling and stomach sagging

Left: example of extreme saddling. Deformation caused by corset-wearing fashions dating back a few years: swayback, semi-swollen and semi-sagging belly in both individuals.

Right: Easy way to observe and identify correct posture, saddling and deformed abdominal lines. Position self against a wall. On the left: normal abdominal and lumbar line. The stomach is hollow, inside of a vertical line drawn from the sternum and no excess fat. On the right: slight saddling. Sagging belly characterized by a lower belly bump.

3) The corset removes all flexibility.

A restricted trunk in a rigid brace cannot, indeed, execute lateral or forward flexion, or backwards extension in a full range of motion.

Women, having their bust "locked", maintain their hips rigid; their trunk mobility is shortened, stuck and the gait is stiff and without grace.

4) The corset destroys general beauty by ways of reduction of physical activity.

Physical activity is just as necessary for the maintenance of beauty as it is for health.

Corsets obviously restrict activity. It is evident that a restrained body is encumbered in it natural movements and cannot perform well. The corseted woman thus carefully avoids any effort; she becomes weak, delicate and lazy physically. The consequences of inactivity, we already know, is always a loss of shapes and curves that is more or less pronounced.

5) In overweight women, the corset produces bizarre effects: it shifts fat deposits and sometimes shifts them to the hips, which then appear huge. [PICS]

# 39. SO-CALLED RATIONAL CORSETS. NATURAL OR MUSCULAR CORSET.

From time to time, we hear of the creation of a new corset model, more rationalized that any preceding models.

Corsets that were trendy twenty years ago used to split the stomach in two. The latest ones do not flatten it, but shrink the lower ribs the same was as their predecessors. Compression is only lateral instead of all-around.

With each new model, so-called medical doctors in seemingly scientific articles, chastise the older versions for causing many disorders and claim new benefits of the latest model, built according to the anatomy of women, and as a grand finale, encourage their female audience to put this beneficial device, which, while giving them a perfect shape, ensures, apparently, the free motion of their internal organs.

All of this would be a joke if health wasn't a consideration at the same time as beauty.

When pointing out the trade-offs of a corset to a women, she hastily responds: "but I am not wearing it too tightly!" not realizing that any compression prevents the proper action of internal organs and encumbers the execution of natural movements. Additionally, if the corset is not too tight in an upright position, we already indicated than when seated, internal organs are always more or less strongly compressed. One needs only try for themselves of this nuisance without seeking additional anatomical or physiological reasons. If corset defenders were forced to wear one, they would quickly change their mind.

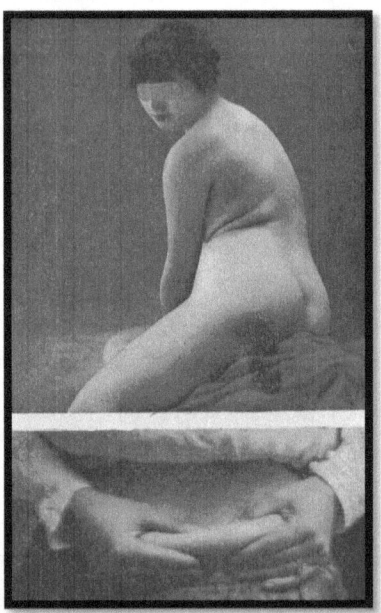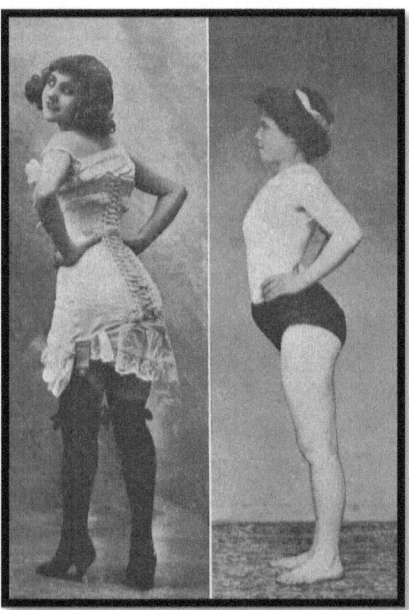

Top: common alteration of the shape as a result of excess fat accumulation. Abnormal fat folds on the flanks. Soft back, no definition, "sausage" arms.

Bottom: Simple way to measure the thickness of fat layers on the abdomen or any other body part: grab between thumb and pointer finger, or first two fingers, the entire layer of fat above the muscles.

CORSET SIDE EFFECTS

Wearing a corset has the effect to increase lumbar curve, to atrophy abdominal muscles, in other words to complete alter the shape of the abs and low back. On the right, the individual shows a "saddled low back" and a sagging belly, despite her bolt upright posture.

There is only one rational corset, that provided by Mother Nature via the abdominal muscles, equally powerful, when developed, as all the scientific or artificial girdling.

Girdles present, to a lesser degree, the same setbacks as true corsets, because they are more or less compressing. As for elastic waistbands, they exercise a *continuous* pressure, very bad for circulation and respiration.

How do you support clothing without cinching the waist, one may ask, since any squeezing is unnatural and the abdominal walls must be *free* for breathing and digestion?

The problem must be solved by having the weight of the clothes supported at the shoulders, not the waist. That's the case for tall dresses.

The most hygienic and esthetic fashions always fulfilled this condition. For instance, the fashions of the First Empire *(France circa 1804-1814)* were merely a modernization of Greek and Roman tunics supported at the shoulders. The waist was only indicated, not squeezed; movements of the abdomen could be freely performed.

In summary, any woman wearing a corset admits her physical weakness. If she were muscular, it would be impossible for her to wear such a device.

The corset, like the bra, should simply belong to the category of orthopedic equipment.

# CHAPTER VIII : BEAUTIFUL OR UGLY POSTURE

## 40. IMPORTANCE OF GOOD POSTURE.

The position that the trunk presents in a natural upright stance, at rest or in motion, constitutes the posture, or the "carry" *(as in how one carries oneself)*.

As a result of the shoulders' mobility, forward or backwards, as well as up and down, and also on the other hand, of the flexibility of the spine forward, backwards and laterally, certain parts of the trunk adopt a variety of habitual stances according to individuals. Some are normal and consequently esthetically pleasing, others are defective, abnormal or non-esthetic.

Nothing is more disgraceful, for instance, than a rounded back, a caved in chest and forward hunched shoulders. These are, nevertheless, fairly common deformations.

It is not enough to be well-proportioned and well-muscled, one needs to bring forward these two elements of beauty with a harmonious way to carry oneself.

A correct posture consists first and foremost in keeping an open chest, maintaining the shoulders back sufficiently, and finally to not hunch the back or drop the neck forward.

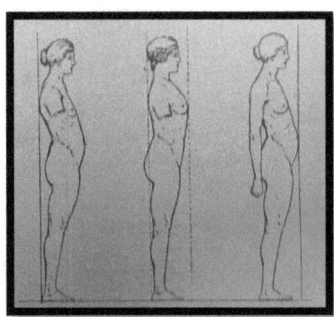

Figure 51. Good and bad posture. Center: Good posture in upright stance. Dotted lines indicate the respective positions of the various body parts in relation to two vertical lines. Facing a wall, only the sternum makes contact. Left: Poor posture. Arched back, protruding belly, caved-in chest, neck forward. Facing a wall, the stomach is in contact instead of the sternum's tip. Back to a wall, the upper back is the only point of contact, along with the heels.

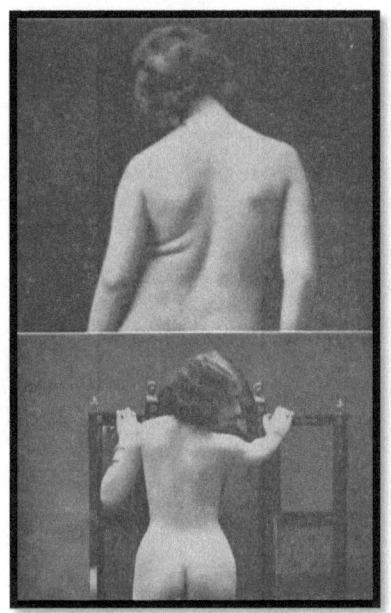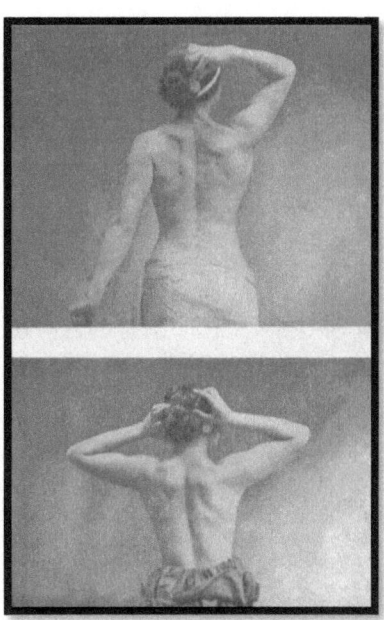

COMPARATIVE STUDY OF THE SHAPE OF THE BACK

Top left panel: common alteration of the back due to excess body fat, localized on the flanks. Abnormal folds. Despite the fat accumulation, the individual presents jutting shoulder blades, indicative of insufficient muscular development.

Bottom left panel: Cylindrical or parallel flanks, resulting from an atrophy of the dorsal muscles.

Right: two remarkable examples of dorsal development (author's students). Note the V-shaped trunk from waist to armpits, resulting from muscular development.

Top right panel: pose exposing the definition of the back muscles (right side especially): trapezius, rear deltoid (right arm) and triceps (left arm).

Bottom right panel: pose emphasizing the development of the sacra-lumbar muscles and the definition of the spinal muscles.

This is of capital importance, not only from a standpoint of esthetics, but also from a hygienic standpoint. It is indispensable, indeed, that the lungs expand freely inside the thoracic cage, in order to develop their full power.

The common poor shape consisting of caving in the chest and round the shoulders forward negatively affect the full expansion of the ribs, and consequently diminishes the amplitude of breathing movements.

When the habitual posture is incorrect, the resulting deformities worsen with age, as a result of a gradual ankylosis of the vertebrae, shoulder joints and ribs; these defects become harder and harder to correct and end up unable to be reversed.

Hence the need to know the principles of correct posture in order to avoid the onset of deformities that we tend to attribute to aging, when they are simply the consequence of bad habits or lack of exercise.

This is especially noticeable when the body is viewed from the side that posture displays its more characteristic aspects. One glance on the trunk from that angle allows to immediately take note of the postural qualities or defects of any individual.

## 41. CAUSES AND DISADVANTAGES OF BAD POSTURE.

The amount of people presenting abnormal or defective posture is considerable in both genders, in all social classes. However, in women, this proportion is greater than in men.

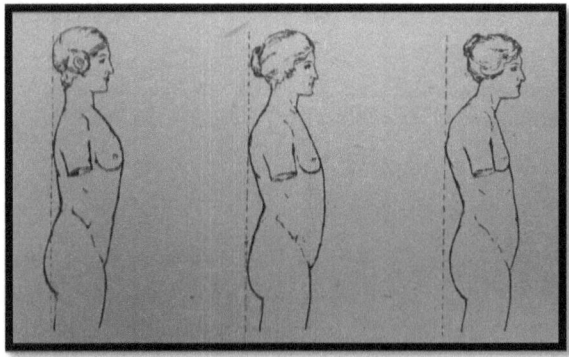

Figure 52. Slouching or rounded back. Left: good posture, open chest, shoulders retracted, neck straight, normal alignment of the back. Center: "let go"/lazy posture. Increased dorsal rounding as a result of neck and chest protraction and rounding of shoulders. Right: settled rounded back. The thorax is flattened, the shoulders are very forward, the chest seems thrown backwards.

This can be due to numerous causes, of which the main ones are:

Firstly, a general muscular atrophy.

The spinal column, poorly supported by the balancing muscles of the trunk, insufficiently developed, collapses either in its upper portion, which causes a hunched back (rounded back), or its lower portion, which results in caving in the lumbar area (sway back), or also laterally, which produces a lateral deviation and lowers one of the shoulders.

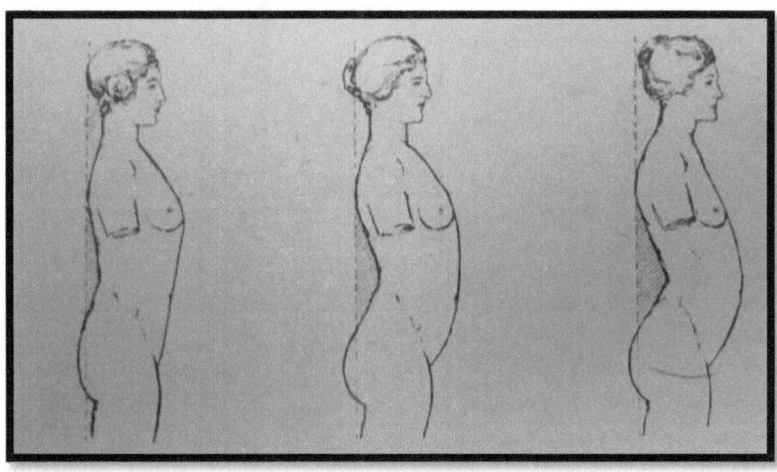

Figure 53: Abnormal and normal lumbar curve. Left: normal lumbar shape, upright trunk, vertical neck axis, open chest. The arching of the low back is slight. Center: slight saddling, increased lumbar curve, the belly is shooting forward slightly. Right: strong saddling, which consequently makes the belly protrude strongly and the low back sways excessively.

On another hand, the shoulder, poorly attached muscularly, protracts under its own weight, which has the resulting effect to cave the chest in and round the back, or it sags and produces dropped shoulders.

When the shoulders are protracted, we can see, on each side of the neck, above the clavicles, two gaps, commonly called "salt shakers", more or less pronounced according to the degree of protraction of the shoulders, or the skinniness of the individual. These gaps disappear as soon as a proper posture is adopted. How many poor women, ignoring this simple detail, have condemned themselves, under the advice of charlatans, to a forced weight gain to fill those darn gaps!

Secondly, habitual nonchalance, careless letting go or laziness in needing to do corrective *straightening* exercises, even when possessing muscles.

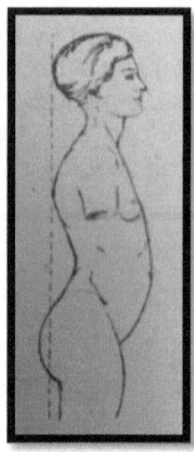

Figure 54. Double saddling: lumbar and cervical. Strong curve in the low back and neck. The chest is caved in and the belly is protruding.

Generally speaking, nearly all movements in a woman's everyday life are done in front of the body in a flexed forward posture, which tends to bring the shoulders forward and to round the back: eating, writing, sewing, lifting objects, ironing, sweeping, playing the piano, etc., etc. It is rare for them to have the need to raise their arms vertically (to reach a high object, to hang by their hands, to throw an object into the air) or forced to maintain an object on top of their head, or to bring their arms behind their shoulders, etc. These are nevertheless natural motions, which have slowly disappeared in ordinary labors of civilized life. We blame their disappearance as a defect or deformity, whenever we cease to perform the movements our body is designed for.

Thirdly, deforming exercises coming from poor training, meaning exercises that pack dysfunction instead of correcting it.

In this category, we must allocated whimsical exercises where they belong, with unnatural equipment: high bar, parallel bars, trapeze, rings, pommel horse etc, practiced in certain women's groups.

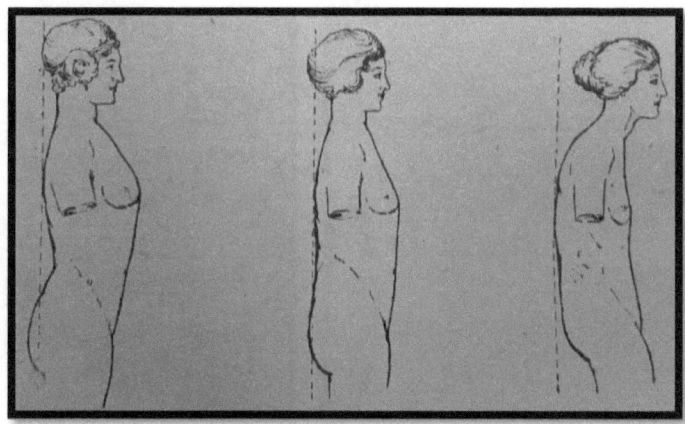

Figure 55. Straight or flat low back. Left: normal lumbar curve. Center: lack of lumbar curve. Right: flat low back with rounded upper back, caved-in chest and forward neck (early kyphosis).

Gymnasts, male or female, practicing on their gymnastics equipment, nearly all have poor posture, because they mostly perform pulling, flexion or tension movements, which tend to bring the shoulders forward, cave the chest in and hunch the back, and never do straightening movements.

Forward trunk or shoulder movements (rounding of the back or neck, shoulder protraction, etc.) are just as natural as backwards extension and straightening movements. But, since the former are performed without the latter being performed, a muscular imbalance in certain areas of the trunk and shoulders occur, which result in the postural deficiencies mentioned earlier.

The natural movements which consist of rounding the neck and the upper back do not represent a hunched posture, which is a consequence of a bad curve in the spine. The examples showing the profile view of the *Venus of Milo* and the person on the left display this point clearly.

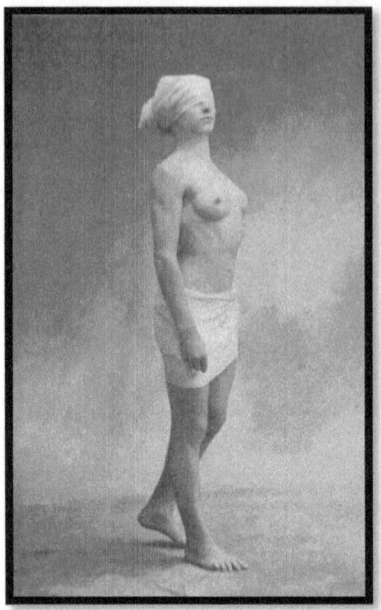
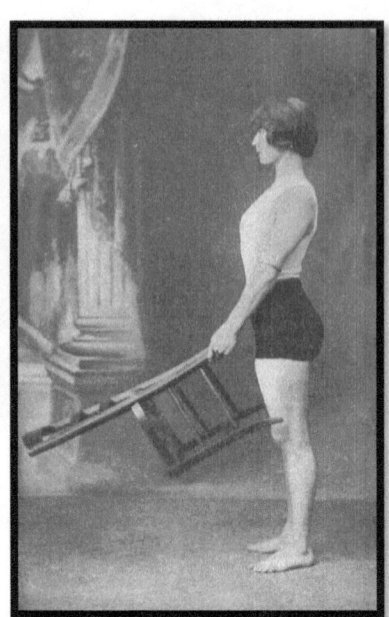

PROPER POSTURE IN UPRIGHT STANCE

Open chest, shoulders retracted, neck vertical and straight, hollow stomach and low back slightly arched.

## 42. CHARACTERISTICS OF CORRECT POSTURE.

In the upright stance, meaning steady on both legs without intentionally leaning the head or the upper body forward, the various portions of the trunk must present a natural profile view in the following way:

- The head is lifted, the chin semi-tucked, the neck is straight and its line is vertical.

- The shoulders are retracted.

- The chest is open, as a result of the retraction of the shoulders, the sternum is projected forward and at an angle of about 45° when the thorax is well developed.

- ◉ The tummy is tucked in relation to the chest; it is inside a vertical line drawn from the tip of the sternum.

- ◉ The low back is slightly arched.

- ◉ From the front, the body is steady on both legs, together and straight, and both shoulders must be level: neither the head nor the trunk are leaning right or left.

When muscular efforts are necessary to adopt this posture, it means the *habitual* stance, during daily activities, is defective. In order to correct it, one must change the way to stand straight when upright, or when seated, then perform forced proper postural movements of corrective exercises until the shoulders maintain themselves backwards naturally, without effort, and the chest remains open.

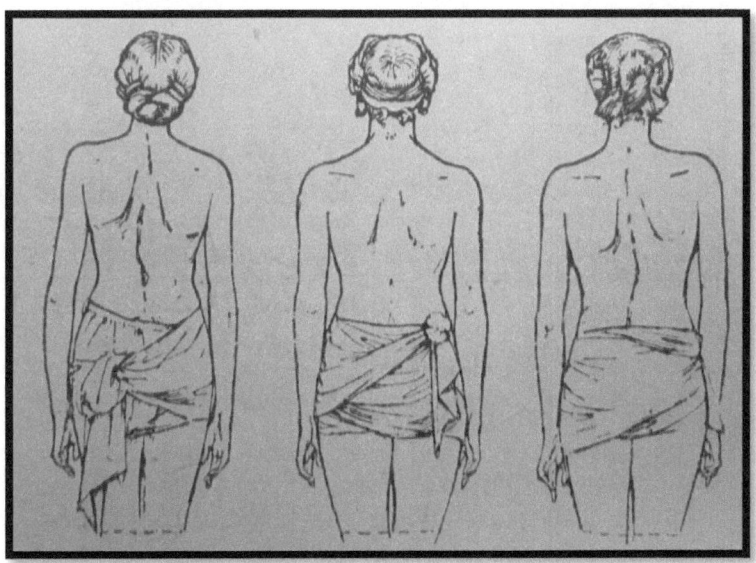

Figure 56. Scoliosis or lateral deformation of the spine. Center: normal straight spine. Left: right scoliosis, right shoulder lower than the left. Right: left scoliosis, left shoulder lower than the right shoulder.

It is important to note that to carry oneself well, outside of some conformation defects impossible to get eradicate, is a matter of *will power* and *good habits*. Performing daily corrective exercises for a few minutes and intensely during training are powerless in totally overcoming a poor posture maintained for the remainder of the day.

To avoid this infamous "rounded back", one must thus, for every day of their existence, be mindful to throw their shoulders backwards and open the chest. In other words, if one gradually becomes nonchalant about it, one may being to hunch slightly, and the day this ugly defect is notice, it is often too late to remedy. Ankylosis has set in and a forced proper stance is insufficient to fight it off.

To remain aware of the body's position and proper posture, one should use the following ways:

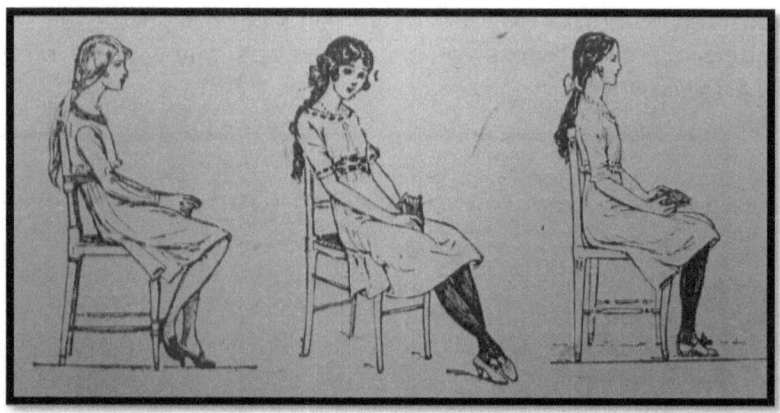

Figure 57. Good and bad posture when seated. Right: goof posture, open chest. Left and center: two bad postures with rounded back, which inevitably lead to a hunching of the back when ongoing and habitual, without being corrected.

1) Back against a wall, the following body parts must be in contact with the wall: heels, calves, buttocks (flattened as needed), back (at shoulder blades level) and the back of the head (hair flat, no bun).

2) Facing a wall, feet together with toes touching the wall or no further than a hand width away, the only part of the body in contact with the wall being the tip of the sternum.

The abdomen is drawn in if no conformation defects or excess fat deposit are added to the assessment of the posture.

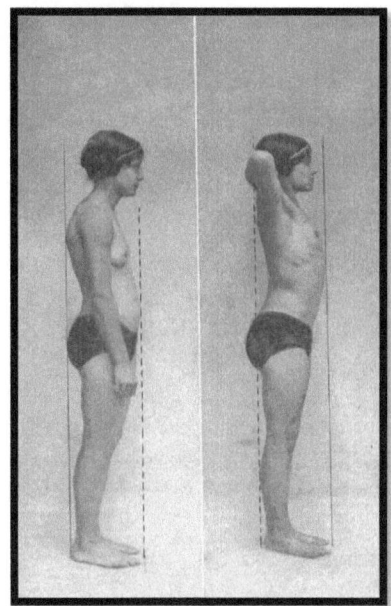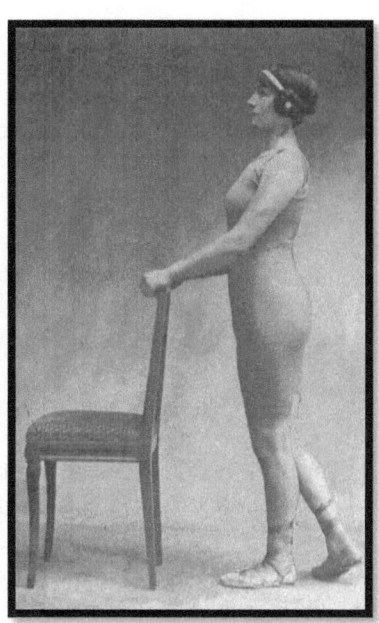

GOOD AND BAD POSTURE IN UPRIGHT STANCE

Left: Lazy posture, caved-in chest, belly forward, neck bent forward, rounded back. This posture, when habitual, rapidly deforms the body and becomes impossible to correct a rounded back or flattening of the thorax. Notice the sagging of the breasts and the "letting go" of the pectoral muscle.

Second from left/center: corrective straightening exercise.

Right: Good posture. Open chest, shoulders back, neck straight, hollow stomach, low back slightly arched.

## 43. CHARACTERISTICS OF INCORRECT POSTURE.

In an upright stance, with the body straight, the following postural defects, when *habitual*, characterize an incorrect posture from a profile view [PIX]:

- ◉ Head tilted forward, chin protruding and lifted.

- ◉ Neck inclined forward, its back line angled instead of being vertical.

- Shoulders forward (strongly forward shoulders are called "coat hangers").

- Chest flat or caved, which give the sternum a faint incline, nearly vertical.

- Stomach protruding forward, extending past the vertical line drawn from the tip of the sternum. This deformity can exist simply as the result of the accumulation of fat around the waist, without necessarily meaning there is poor posture, or being considered a result of such.

- Overly pronounced curve at the cervical spine and top part of thoracic spine, causing a hunching of the back, commonly referred to as rounded back, or generalized curve in the entire back, the low back, the neck, causing kyphosis.

- Excessive curvature of the lumbar spine, causing saddling or lordosis, a frequent deformity. Or, on the contrary, a flat or straight low back, meaning with too weak an arch or without one.

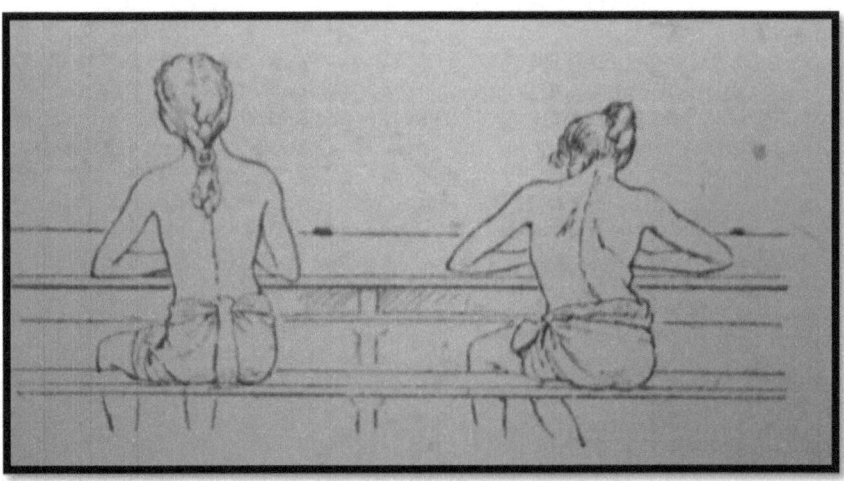

Figure 58. Good and bad posture when seated. Left: good posture, the spine is straight. Right: bad posture, common among school children. The spine is deviated. Maintaining this posture for hours daily can rapidly produce scoliosis.

From front or side, the defects characterizing a poor posture are:

- ◉ Head or trunk tilting right or left, or with one shoulder higher than the other.

- ◉ Lateral curve of the dorsal vertebrae, having as a result a deviation called scoliosis

All these deviations can exist both in women as in men to various degrees. In general, the saddling as for forced consequence a rounded back, and the rounded back determines the degree of protrusion of the belly. Scoliosis drops one of the shoulders.

These defective repercussions have the effect of imbalancing the pieces of the skeleton, destroyed by the abnormal shape of some of these parts.

# ABOUT THE AUTHOR

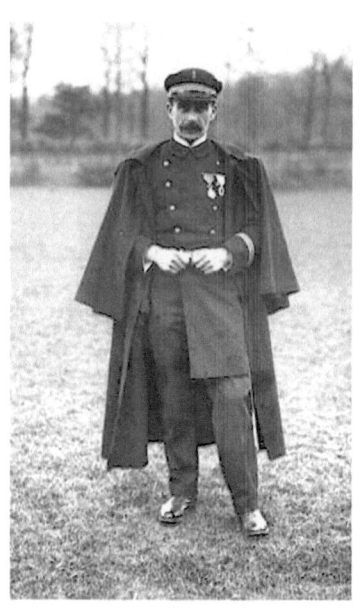

**Georges Hébert** (27 April 1875 – 2 August 1957) was a pioneering French physical educator, theorist and instructor. He believed that athletic skill must be combined with courage and altruism. He eventually developed this ethos into his personal motto, "Être fort pour être utile" ("Being strong to be useful"). In 1955, at the 50th birthday of the Natural Method, Hébert was named Commander of the Legion of Honor by the French government in recognition of his many services to his country. In 1957, George Hébert, by then suffering from general paralysis, cultivated the admiration of his entourage by relearning how to walk, speak and write. He died on August 2 of that year in Tourgéville, Calvados. Hébert's teachings have been an important influence on the emergence of Parkour as a training discipline in its own right.

# ABOUT THE TRANSLATOR

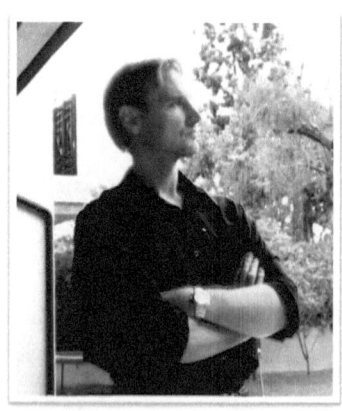

Philippe Til, né Philippe Til Tomaszewski of Polish parents, raised in France until he came to the USA for college, is a multi-faceted fitness entrepreneur whose journey took him from training clients of all levels and professions, to having his own studio, writing content for various fitness companies and organizations and now adapting historical fitness books. At the urge of one of his mentors, Dr Ed Thomas, he took it upon himself to translate and adapt the works of his fellow Frenchman Georges Hébert, whose fitness explorations in The Natural Method (La Méthode Naturelle) book series provide the historical basis for many of today's training methodologies, whether they are aware of it or not!

www.ingramcontent.com/pod-product-compliance
Lightning Source LLC
Chambersburg PA
CBHW020900310526
45786CB00018B/490